BITE ME!
CHANGE YOUR LIFE
ONE BITE AT A TIME

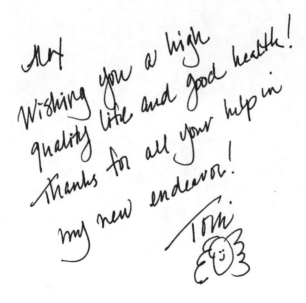

BITE ME!

CHANGE YOUR LIFE
ONE BITE AT A TIME

*An Inspirational Journey of
Re-Invention to a Sustainable,
Healthy Lifestyle.*

Toni Julian

authorHOUSE®

AuthorHouse™
1663 Liberty Drive
Bloomington, IN 47403
www.authorhouse.com
Phone: 1-800-839-8640

First published by AuthorHouse   06/28/2011

ISBN: 978-1-4634-1938-7 (sc)
ISBN: 978-1-4634-1937-0 (dj)
ISBN: 978-1-4634-1936-3 (ebk)

Library of Congress Control Number: 2011909598

Printed in the United States of America

Any people depicted in stock imagery provided by Thinkstock are models, and such images are being used for illustrative purposes only.

Certain stock imagery © Thinkstock.

This book is printed on acid-free paper.

Because of the dynamic nature of the Internet, any web addresses or links contained in this book may have changed since publication and may no longer be valid. The views expressed in this work are solely those of the author and do not necessarily reflect the views of the publisher, and the publisher hereby disclaims any responsibility for them.

COVER CREDITS

Photography: Jim Nelson Photography
Hair Stylist: Patti Keating, Owner, City Savvy Salon in Campbell, CA
Make-up: Kathy Obot, Owner, Kase' Cosmetics
Proofreading and Editing: Valerie Marie Kohl

NOTICE

Mention of specific companies, organizations, brands or authorities in this book does not imply endorsement by the publisher or author, nor does mention of specific companies, organizations or authorities imply they endorse this book.

The brand name products mentioned in this book are trademarks or registered trademarks of their respective companies. The author, publisher, manufacturers, or distributors cannot accept legal responsibility for any problem arising out of the use of or experimentation with the methods described.

Nutritional information for all brand name products mentioned in this book was provided by their companies or on official nutrition labels. Those who do not provide complete nutrition information to the public, the estimates for their products were obtained from CalorieKing.com, an independent nutrition information and communication service that is owned and operated by Family Health Publications Pty Ltd. Nutrition information noted for each recipe was derived through using the bodybugg® or Exerspy, calorie and nutrient tracking online software services owned by Apex Fitness and DotFit, respectively.

IMPORTANT:

This book is not intended as a substitute for the medical and nutritional advice from physicians. Consult a physician before starting any new diet or exercise regimen and regularly consult a physician in all matters relating to his or her health, and particularly with respect to any symptoms that may require diagnosis or medical attention. Content provided in this book is based on the opinion and experiences of the author and does not take the place of medical and nutritional advice.

CONTENTS PAGE

DEDICATION

To my angel, Barbara Wyman-Sun, 1959-2007, who's courageous will and free spirit, moved me to help others.

INTRODUCTION

In earlier years, I would lay in bed attempting to drift into a hopefully deep slumber. My body felt like it would take ten years of sleep to recover from my full day. I had reoccurring dreams that I am running; running through the streets in slow motion, struggling to round the curb. No matter how much effort I exerted, I would gain only a few inches. I could never catch up. I would never make progress. After years of these reoccurring dreams, with unsettled and slightly tortured feelings, a slow realization came into focus, like a low resolution, grainy and highly pixilated photograph, once indiscernible, now pixel by pixel creating a crisp picture I can now recognize. I would never truly feel well; never be able to figuratively run unencumbered if I didn't make some lifestyle changes, and *now*.

This gradual confrontation of the truth is that we, as a collective of individuals are solely responsible what I call the "American de-condition". It is a well-documented fact that nearly 70% of all Americans are either overweight or obese, one of the leading contributors to a proliferation of medical issues. A very small percent of our population, perhaps 10%, can actually be considered "fit". The rest of have allowed ourselves to become out of shape, nutritionally deprived and prone to disease, weight issues, hormonal imbalances, and injury. We become tired, depressed, and depleted, and in some cases become a burden on our families and a proverbial weight on the back of an already dysfunctional health care system, yet most of us haven't taken the action necessary to resolve the problem.

America's de-conditioned state is compounded by our procrastination and general lack of motivation. We all know the statistics, we hear them frequently; they don't necessarily move us to take the initiative for change. Are we expecting someone to fix the problem or waiting for some in-your-face, life-altering experience which threatens our very existence before taking action? We want an instant fix; fruit and vegetables in a pill, a miracle drink or foods mailed to our doorsteps. Perhaps the FDA can provide increased regulation for the proliferation of deceptive food labeling cases. Must we wait until we have diabetes, high blood pressure and heart disease? The bottom line is we all have the opportunity to be healthy, in addition to the freedom to let ourselves go. Only we are accountable for ourselves. Our personal passivity and demand for convenience are our own worst enemies.

Inexcusably, we have passed down our sedentary lifestyles and poor eating habits to our children. We allow our children to eat the most convenient and lowest quality foods possible. They grow up thinking a tomato slice on their fast food burger is a "serving of vegetables" and nothing tastes good if it's not dripping with sugar and fat. High cholesterol, obesity, early onset diabetes and hip and joint issues, once considered diseases of our older populations are unfortunately now bestowed upon our children at alarming rates. Further confirming our lackadaisical attitude toward our health, over half our dogs and cats are overweight or obese. Certainly our furry friends are not raiding the treat jar late at night by themselves.

Many of us have the desire to learn how to shift thinking toward better health only to be confronted by external influences providing confusing, and often conflicting, information. Everywhere I turn I am bombarded with confusing messages: From pharmaceutical companies, to food manufacturers and marketers, weight loss companies, and fast food providers; from friends offering well-meaning advice to our respected physicians who take stewardship of our collective health to the best of their ability.

I love humankind, I love my family, my neighbors and my friends, and I love the friends I have not yet met. With this in the forefront of my mind, I carry a deep sadness and disappointment as I am confronted by "misinformation" as well as an intense anger in situations when I know we are being intentionally misled.

My belief is that prevention is the answer and that lies only within our self. We must change our eating habits, as well as our lifestyle, in a way that makes our newly-learned, healthy behaviors SUSTAINABLE. Become role models and our children will do as we do.

We have an unprecedented opportunity here to change our lives, our family's lives, the lives within our community, and beyond. We need education, accountability, and most of all, hope. We must educate ourselves to make the best choices in support of our wellbeing. We must be accountable to ourselves and to the one body we are given on this Earth, as well as those in our inner circle—the people we affect for better or worse—depending upon our level of wellness. Let's have hope so that we may become empowered and not allow our minds and bodies to degrade to the point of ultimate defeat.

It is never too late to start to help yourself and those around you. We can accomplish this empowerment ourselves and ultimately change one life at a time. I am walking proof of that. I've been through most everything life can throw at me, and at over 50 dealing with the added complexities of aging as well.

> *"I am on a personal and professional mission to defend the right of people to eat well and to motivate them to shift their thinking toward better health."*

This passion to help others was born out of the loss of my best friend to Pancreatic Cancer, as well as my own serious medical issues just a few short years ago. I quite literally can say "I stake my life" on the assertion that lifestyle changes WORK, because I am a living example. My personal story is bared to all in its vulnerability, from misfortune to fulfillment and everything in between, in hopes that you may find inspiration and motivation to help shift your thinking toward a healthier lifestyle.

My goal is to inspire you to raise your personal nutrition bar, so I will be sharing what I've learned as a full-time working mom of four, who has endeavored on a journey to a sustainable, healthy lifestyle, as well as changed careers to a Lifestyle and Certified Nutrition Coach, Figure Competitor and NASM Certified Personal Trainer.

You may have noticed I do not have a forward written by a physician to lend credibility to my words, as you may see frequently in other self-help, diet or fitness books. I did not have a staff of researchers, writers, editors, photographers and designers, nor did I have professional chefs or a test kitchen at my disposal. I am not married to a publisher or have unlimited resources. This book is boot-strapped from my heart in all authenticity, so that in your dreams, you will not have to run in slow motion around those curbs feeling frustration at not making progress toward your well being. I hope to help you to sprint around them feeling light and strong, knowing you are giving your best to make a difference—not only in your life but helping others learn to take impeccable care as well. Feeling good is contagious and looking good is pure inspiration.

May you find the tools and motivation you need to change your life one bite at a time!

Toni Julian

CHAPTER 1

ONE BITE AT A TIME

"The greatest wealth a man may acquire is the wisdom he gains from living. And sometimes out of small beginnings come the forces that shape a whole life."

~John Tucker Battle, Screen Writer

You can change your life one bite at a time, one meal at a time, and one day at a time, just by making simple changes in your diet and lifestyle. Eventually all those good choices add up to a better lifestyle and quality of life; one with increased energy, a leaner body, an improved immune system and happier outlook.

What we eat, where we eat, and how much we eat is entirely our decision. It is through the choices we make on a daily basis that have the most significant impact on how we look and feel. Unfortunately, the majority of Americans are misled and left at the mercy of whatever information is conveniently accessible, which is ironically how most of us eat; whatever is convenient and accessible. The quality of this information is as poor as the quality of our food.

We need to regroup; get back to a common sense approach about our nutrition because the way we look and feel is largely impacted by what we eat. And frankly, dining at most restaurants, or buying processed, prepared or fast foods puts us at a disadvantage. Even with the new nutrient disclosure laws, we often do not know the quality of ingredients used or if the information is even accurate. Portion size is yet another issue. Food labeling can be intentionally misleading, and going on diets where the foods are provided or fad diets where certain food types are restricted may be helpful short term, but only while you strictly adhere to them, and they won't teach you how to make choices for yourself that are sustainable. An astonishing 95% of people who attempt fad diets gain their weight back within the first year.

The better alternative: Learn how to build a strong nutritional foundation; eat in a life-smart way that balances your blood sugar, helps stave off disease and puts you in a better position to persevere through illness, stress and whatever else life happens to throw your way.

Make simple, wholesome meals for yourself and your family, and you will see the benefits within a short time. You will be introduced to the concept of "clean eating" in the next chapter, and if you read on, you'll be enlightened to learn how to apply simple guidelines to your life so these healthy eating habits will be sustainable, for the rest of your life. You will begin to feel phenomenal, and your family won't realize they are eating so much healthier. Think about the positive role model you will be setting for your children; leading by example. Start making good choices now. It's really never too late to start making positive changes and it's not as difficult as you think. You can still eat the foods you love in moderation and you won't need to make changes you're not ready for.

Our ancestors lived their lives more moderately. In America, just 150 years ago, men, women and children lived challenging lives. Women needed to eat about 4000 calories each day just to provide them with energy to get through their agrarian day; working the fields, cooking, washing, and tending to their families. Present day, we live an over-abundant lifestyle, to the point that we need to create ways to expend our excess energy. To put it very simply, we eat too much and move too little. Even 50 years ago lifestyles were better calorically balanced. We need to learn how to eat like our grandparents, not our parents, who began to incorporate highly processed, convenient foods into their diets.

Anyone who knows me has heard me brag about my family. My Grandmother, Nancy, is 102 today as I write. Although I grew up geographically distanced from her, even as a young child I watched her with an intense curiosity. She is a feisty and petite Italian with beautiful skin, white teeth and a propensity for waking you up by throwing a shoe at your head. Just ask my father.

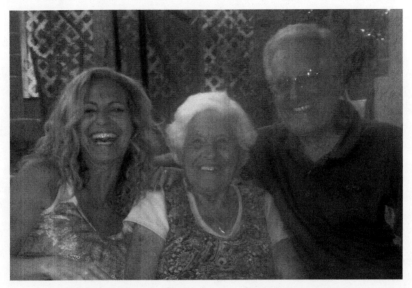

Three generations of Julian's; Grandma Nancy at 102 in center with son John at right and Granddaughter, Toni at left.

What I remember most about her is her lifestyle, which may be a strange thing for a kid to notice. She was different from my parents, from the "old world" with a heavy Italian accent and unrefined ways. Every day she walked for a miles touring the neighborhood, picking mustard greens from nearby fields for dinner. While it's one thing to pick a neighbor's weeds—I realized early she was completely oblivious of neighborly etiquette—when she came home with bunches of roses from their garden too. She made her own pasta from scratch, using a fork to pinch the edges of the ravioli together. A typical Italian, she never measured ingredients and the kitchen was coated with a dusting of flour. For dessert she would slice fresh oranges and put them on the table. All her foods were whole. She bought little that had a nutrition

3

facts label attached to it. It came from the Earth, and embarrassingly I learned, at times from the neighbor's front yard.

We are the new centurions if we play our cards right, we too will live to be 100 like my grandmother. Although to me it's not so much the length of life we lead as much as the quality in which we live it, which makes it vitally important to shift the way we think about our eating and fitness habits while we have the opportunity and work toward not only extending our lives but the quality of our life as well.

You will learn how to make lifestyle changes, while eating the foods you love, in a way that is simple and convenient. You will be walked through the process of learning how you metabolize foods and how to reset your own metabolism. You will be motivated and encouraged, and most of all finally see the rewards from your efforts. So let's get started on our journey together!

CHAPTER 2

TONI'S STORY OF REINVENTION

"My main goal is to inspire you to take impeccable care of yourself. I have proven it is never too late to start."
— *Toni Julian*

It took a while for me to understand the benefits of being proactive with my health. I learned the hard way; I am hoping you will not have to repeat my mistakes. Whether you're a teacher, an engineer, a firefighter or a busy parent, why not be at the top of your game? We're always "on" and spending our days not feeling as well as we can, takes away a part of our gift of life and erodes our happiness. Not every ailment or disease is preventable, but why gamble? At a minimum, improve the quality of your life so you are in the best position to get through whatever life throws at you.

Essentially, I've experienced a full and diverse life; from the joyfulness of love and marriage and babies, to the challenges of illnesses, divorce, hospitalizations, horrific car accidents and permanent injuries, while juggling a business and blending a family.

I'd like now to share my story with you, a story of healing, of self-improvement, and of stretching well beyond the confines of the routine of my predictable daily life, in hopes that you may relate to at least parts of it.

5

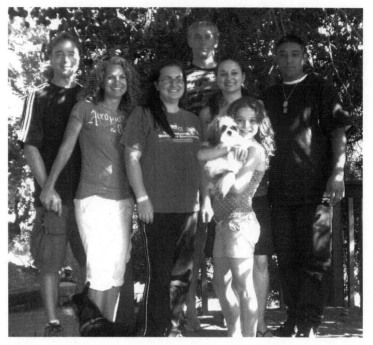

My Family

I was the typical mom, striving to maintain that delicate balance between being a full time working mother; having a full time career and blending a new family in a dynamic household with a husband and four kids; a "yours, mine and ours" family, including our new infant and three elementary age kids. I taught art in their classrooms and was a "room mom" for years. I juggled soccer practices and Girl Scout cookie sales, made Halloween outfits and had home cooked meals on the table every night. Eventually, our three older kids were in high school, and heading into college to explore new-found freedoms in different parts of the country.

After spending decades in the corporate world—I had several businesses, one of which was a Marketing Communications firm where we provided trade show, conference and special event program management services to a host of technology companies in Silicon Valley—as well as an Interior Design Firm—finding balance between taking care of myself, and all the other demands of family life, were beginning to take its toll.

Although I thought I took good care of myself—I ate reasonably well, healthier than most, worked out at a local gym, and was very active, it wasn't enough. I didn't feel well most of the time, and more often than not felt "under the weather." When my life was not in balance, say I was a little sleep deprived, maybe didn't eat as well as I could and it was "that time of the month," my husband would joke with me about it being the "perfect storm." My temperament was so delicate; I'd get hit with a massive migraine if I couldn't keep all elements of my life in balance.

Being afflicted with frequent migraines and chronic lower back pain, from multiple rear-end collisions, a skydiving accident and a near-death car accident in my twenties, the cumulative effect was debilitating. If I tripped on a curb, I was so de-conditioned, I was sure to throw my back out. When our youngest daughter was eight weeks old, I happened to sneeze while holding her and dropped to the floor, completely blowing out my back. Fortunately, I had the wherewithal to gently place her on the bed before I crumpled into a heap on the floor, then crawled to the phone for help. I found myself in bed for nine days with a cooler of yogurt and diet drinks to sustain me while my husband was at work. I began participating in physical therapy, but it wasn't enough and more importantly, it made me feel old and like an invalid!

Waking up to coffee in the morning, diet Pepsi's and a Lean Cuisine at lunch, and winding down at night over a bottle of wine shared with my husband, I did not realize I was self-medicating to overcome the stress, the lack of energy, the exhaustion, and the anxiety of the challenges that can (and did) come along while blending our families in a healthy way. I was on medications for the migraines, the anxiety and situational depression, and felt just like a bottle of 7up that's been sitting out open for a week . . . flat!

In spite of these challenges, I always looked on the upside. I felt happy, blessed and appreciative for all I had going in my life. But honestly, something had to give, it was no longer working for me, but I had difficulty envisioning being able to make the necessary changes. It just seemed too overwhelming and I was so close to the tree all I could see was the bark, rather than the composite of beautiful branches and leaves called my life. I was not enjoying my life the way I knew I wanted to.

The Wake-up Call

I didn't fully come to the realization that I had really bitten it, until I was given a harsh wake-up call. That epiphany came with the death of my best friend, Barbara Wyman-Sun, in the summer of 2007. We had been friends since we were 11 years old, nearly 40 years, and we lead parallel lives both being pregnant with our respective youngest children. Barb was an amazing mother; she didn't just have a refrigerator to showcase her kid's art work, she dedicated an entire kitchen wall. She knew how to have fun and loved being silly, regardless of what other people thought. I still remember her birthday, sitting on a throne on her front lawn with a crown and a robe, surrounded by her subjects (friends). I admired her being so authentic and unique. Sadly, Barb was diagnosed with Pancreatic Cancer at the age of 48 and through my research learned there was only a 1% chance of survivability after one year. I kept telling her, "Barb, that one percent can be YOU!"

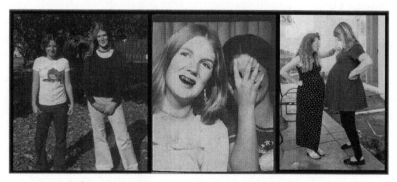

From left to right: Toni and Barb in their freshman year of high school. A photo booth shot (Toni is the shy one on the right). A candid picture of Barb and Toni pregnant with their last born children, taken by Barb's mom, Beth.

Feeling powerless to help, I went to church for the first time in 30 years. I was prompted to pray for a miraculous recovery for my friend. I felt there was something I needed to learn from this situation and also felt certain I would gain some important help. The take-away was two strong messages I knew I was meant to hear. First, use your skills to help those around you, and the second was to live your life with grace. Don't ask for life to easy, because it isn't; ask God to learn how to live it gracefully.

At the same time I was also diagnosed with high-risk cervical dysplasia (CIN1) and underwent surgery to hopefully prevent the spread of full-blown uterine cancer. I was unaware of this dormant virus until my immune system became compromised and unleashed the disease. I would go to bed at night with tears streaming down my cheeks, thinking "How could this be, we have four kids?" One of my other closest friends, Jan, had shared with me that she had been diagnosed with the exact disease many years earlier, and within nine months had developed into ovarian cancer and hemorrhaged after surgery. She is fortunate to have survived it. I was terrified.

JOURNAL ENTRY 3/23/07

"A few days ago I was diagnosed with CIN1, Cervical Intraepithelial Neoplasia. I was told I had been infected with HPV, and that it is the high risk type virus that can lead to full-blown cervical cancer if left untreated. Part of me wants to sound clinical but the other part of me has tears streaming down my cheeks as I write. It's 12:39AM and I can't sleep. I close my eyes and the most extreme and dark thoughts go through my mind and I am ashamed I have invited them."

Given my friends deteriorating condition, I could not even tell her I was sick. Within a couple of days of my discovery, I was honored to be asked by her family to help with her care after they set her up in a hospital bed at home so she could be closest to those that loved her. I brought cookie dough, cutters and colorful sprinkles and spent some time with her kids, baking in the kitchen. I was so very blessed to be with her, to have an opportunity to talk with her albeit briefly. I didn't know if she was lucid, but I told her I loved her and thanked her for helping me through my difficult high school years (that you will learn about later) in hopes that my words and feelings would be heard. The next day, after a 17 month battle, she left a devastated husband, two kids and loving parents behind. Out of respect for the family, I am omitting the private details.

My husband and I had previously planned a trip to Italy and were on a plane the very next day. I could not stop the steady stream of tears and my despair plunged even deeper when I realized I would miss her funeral the following week. Feeling guilty and trapped so far away from home, I decided to pay respects to her in my own way by going into every church I encountered in every city we visited and decided to say a few words for her in the less popular, restricted areas for prayer, while thousands of tourists flocked the halls of the basilicas in Florence, Venice, Sorrento, Cinque Terre and Rome. A sense of levity had settled in my soul as I felt her presence and was comforted—knowing she was with God—and whispered a silent commitment to help others, although it was not clear in what way at the time.

With the loss of this beautiful long-time friend, combined with experiencing the tumultuous emotions of the unpredictability of my own medical condition, I was forced to assess my mortality as well as question whether I had done all I could for my friend. Pangs of guilt passed through me as I asked myself what caused her to pass at such a young age. Was there something I could have done to help prevent this disease? Could it have been related to her diet or the excess "baby weight" as she called it, that she carried around her middle? Her physicians said she was "unlucky." Although this provided no answer to the questions I pondered, I knew in my heart it was time to raise my personal wellness bar and reach out to help others to do the same.

It was the motivation I needed to make lifestyle changes and begin to reinvent myself. It was time. I came through it when my friend didn't and I was determined to make something good come from the loss. My conviction was further reinforced as my awareness of the plight of those around me, and I began to delve into what I call "the American de-condition," or gradual loss of our wellness and fitness conditioning in this country.

At the time I wish I had someone to walk me through the process of making lifestyle changes, I honestly don't think I even knew what to call the journey I was embarking upon. I'm writing this so hopefully you can relate to at least some parts of my story, and take the proactive road I wish I had taken by making incremental changes now; to make lifestyle changes before you really have to or are forced to learn the consequences of your inactions.

The Real Journey Begins

The overwhelming majority of how we look and feel is based on nutrition, so I focused on changing my eating regimen first, and made gradual changes over time, changes that I could handle and incorporate into my busy lifestyle. Although I am a disciplined person, I knew I would set myself up to fail if I attempted to make all the necessary changes at once.

I looked at each day as one bite at a time, one meal at a time. Making good choices the best I could, reading everything educational I could get my hands on, (I even earned a personal training certification from NASM, the National Academy of Sports Medicine, and just recently, a nutrition coaching certification from the IBNFC) so I could thoroughly understand how to transform my body and most importantly, my health.

Life-Smart Changes and My Family

The most significant impact came in how and what I ate. I put a great deal of emphasis on developing healthy recipes over the last several years, and being a busy full-time, entrepreneurial working mom, discovered meal solutions to leverage my time in the kitchen.

A critical component of all this is that we have a large family, my husband loves spicy foods, our youngest daughter has many food allergies, and our oldest daughter has Celiac Disease, a toxic reaction to gluten (the protein found in wheat). In addition, my regimen demanded that the food be nutritious and above all, delicious! So many different needs to meet, what a challenge!

I found I could satisfy everyone by making foods in a "life smart" way. That is, to make healthy foods my new "convenience" foods; making them as accessible as a drive-through on a regular basis. Being able to freeze them, take them along on snacks, pre-portion the meals, and provide an ideal balance of protein, carbohydrates and healthy fats, all these strategies became tools I could use. This was my life, it was real, and it required real solutions.

The benefits to our family were surprisingly substantial. When beginning this, I did not realize the extent of the positive impact it would have on us. I could begin to see the changes in my body and my energy level; however I was surprised when my husband mentioned during dinner that he had unintentionally dropped 10 pounds without realizing it (incidentally, he did not need to). He attributed it to the modifications in the dinners I was preparing as he had not made any other changes to his eating regimen.

The other significant difference is in our children; our youngest daughter is so aware of what she is eating and is now also proud of her fitness abilities. She asks me questions like, "How much protein do I need each day?" and is beginning to read food labels. How many 10 year olds ask, "How much fat is in this?" She is also becoming acutely aware of how she feels when she eats certain foods, knowing she is feeling well normally, and is miserable after making unhealthy choices.

As a strong-willed, determined and bright young girl, she often asserts her position and shows immense persistence. We know this will serve her well later in life although there are times when a flippant attitude just plain tests my patience. With our other children, the disciplinary action included sending them to their room so they would have time to think through their actions and realize how wrong they were (wink wink). By the fourth child, I realized the total ridiculousness of this and as I embarked on my health and fitness journey asked how will this change her attitude? What is the benefit of allowing a child to hang out in their room and play with their toys, read their books and have quiet time while I stew downstairs? Seriously, I wanted to be sent to *my* room, it sounded like fun to me. I decided to try something new that was much more useful. I always believed kids should voice their opinions, but in a respectful way. If this was not the case, I would tell her to "Drop and give me ten!"—push-ups that is—and of course she would respond with an indignant "Really? Mom, really?" So I'd ratchet it up a notch:

"15."
Eye roll.
"20."
"Mom! You can't make me do this!"
"25."

Eventually we would both start laughing, giving the situation a little levity; and she would eek out her pushups, proud of herself for her accomplishment. To that end she just placed second at school during fitness assessments, the true bonus.

Our oldest daughter was impacted in a positive way as well. She had been living with undiagnosed Celiac disease since she was five, which had evolved into toxic food-poisoning-like symptoms that left her severely ill in her early 20's. In college, her grades plummeted and she was rarely well enough to work. Living in Ohio, she had fallen into poor quality eating habits leaving her overweight, hormonally imbalanced and acutely ill most days of the week. I flew her back home to finally glean diagnoses from her physicians. (Although we had her tested and evaluated by several doctors over the years, Celiac disease was mostly unknown; in fact only 5% of all cases in the U.S. have been diagnosed currently in the U.S. There is no pharmacological solution to Celiac Disease, making research highly unappealing to the pharmaceutical industry when the only cure is eating natural, healthy, gluten-free foods.) In spite of inconclusive test results, we were keenly aware of the effects of gluten and the toll it had taken on her quality of life. We worked together and developed a new, healthy eating plan, free of gluten and she set off on a new direction. After a week she stepped on the bathroom scale to check her progress as far as weight was concerned.

I heard a loud "clunk" and ran to her side. She was so surprised she had literally fallen off the scale! Rather than being in a toxic, inflammatory state, her body shifted into better balance; she had lost five pounds. Ongoing adoption of these habits yielded her a 30 pound reduction in a matter of months and a return to her normal weight within a year. Her efforts toward making lifestyle changes and gluten-free choices turned her life around. She feels well most of time and can manage her health purely through proper nutrition. On a side note, some people assume that eating "gluten free" equates to instant weight reduction and improved health. Many G-free foods on the market are loaded with fat and sugar. If removing gluten from your diet makes you feel better, then by all means, do it and replace it with whole foods, not processed, fad "food-like" substances that masquerade as a healthy option.

And our son, that is another story. He has an aversion to eating anything green, unless it's Jell-o. That rules out most vegetables, but perhaps someday he will find it important to eat more balanced.

The Three Month Transformation

On the fitness side, I invested in a personal trainer, Adam, who made all the difference in keeping me focused and helped me understand how to maximize my workouts.

A contest was held at my gym; the goal being to lose the most body fat and gain the most muscle mass over an eight-week period. I thought I didn't have a chance in the world, because in my mind I wasn't really overweight, but I went for it anyway. I experimented with foods and became painfully aware of my poor eating (and drinking) habits. It was astounding what the right foods combined with resistance training can do. I began to feel better as each week progressed and as I became stronger, my back pain and migraines were minimized. My hormone levels became more balanced, as did my moods, and my night time "hot flashes" became a thing of the past.

I started out at 5' 3", 124 lbs and 28% body fat, which I learned is called "skinny-fat" (a healthy range for women is between 20 to 24%). I had never heard of that phenomenon. It means we have very little lean muscle mass proportionately, and even though we may be small, we have a high percentage of fat. I had little strength or energy. In fact, I look back now and think about the "girlie pushups" off my knees and barely being able to do 10 of them when I first started my training program. (When I hit my 50th birthday I popped out 50 dynamic pushups off my toes—no problem.)

My metabolism seemed slow, I typically ate between 1000 and 1400 calories a day and felt I was gaining weight on such a small amount of food. When we intake so few calories, our body goes into a hoarding preservation mode and doesn't want to lose the fat, so my trainer suggested I bump up my calories. That made no sense, but he was right. Increasing my calories slightly allowed me to gain muscle, which in turn increased my metabolism.

After I made the adjustments, I had lost 14 pounds of fat and gained 6 pounds of muscle, down 10 points from 28% to 18% body fat and leveled out at 116 pounds in EIGHT weeks. Much to my surprise, I won the contest, and 10 free training sessions.

Within three months, I really started to notice major changes. My body was lean and I was feeling much better. I supercharged my metabolism by letting go of all the misconceptions and information I thought I knew about eating.

The Ultimate Challenge

> "It's my life, it's now or never. I ain't gonna live forever; I just want to live while I'm alive"
>
> -It's My Life Lyrics by Bon Jovi

After eight months, my trainer suggested I enter a natural body-building contest. I had difficulty exposing myself in a bikini at the beach, how would I stand before hundreds in a posing suit that could fit inside a matchbox? I was so far out of my comfort zone, but wanted to meet the challenge.

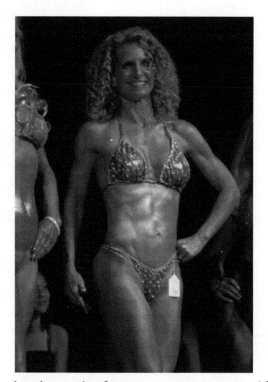

After only eight months of starting my new nutrition and fitness regimen, I tied for first place (and took second) in the ABA/INBA Bay Area Natural Sports Model Open competition. An "open" competition means competing against all age groups starting in the 20's.

The competition was an amazing experience. I felt that just being there was a blessing. Being fit and healthy is a gift. Figure competitions are not for everyone, we don't all want or even need to do this; it was a personal goal and challenge, a way to keep me on track and focused. This experience validated my conviction that my life should be built on unique experiences that add richness and value. We only grow by stretching ourselves, and that sometimes means putting ourselves in situations that make us uncomfortable. It also means being open-minded and allowing ourselves to be introspective, to not be fearful of change and to let go of something when it isn't working for you. If it doesn't serve you, lose it.

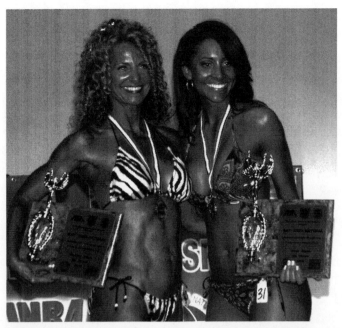

After one year: posing with my 20-something beautiful friend Grace (on right) during the Bay Area Natural Open Figure Competition. I placed second overall.

Sustainability and a Test of Fortitude

Having built a strong nutrition and lifestyle foundation has proven to be invaluable. My eating and fitness habits, modified incrementally over time are sustainable because the changes were not based on deprivation; therefore I had the ability to be consistent, rather than set myself up for failure. After three years of living my new sustainable lifestyle, my body fat is at 18% and my weight a healthy 124. Being a work in progress, I have continued to increase my muscle mass and in turn, raise my metabolism. I now have a strong immune system; I can't think of the last time I had a cold or the flu.

The benefit of being proactive and laying this strong lifestyle foundation has served me well this last year especially. What I didn't realize when I began this journey, is that previous injuries, combined with the added complexity of aging would test my fortitude with such vengeance.

Just this last summer of 2010, I went from thriving to being unable to walk more than a few minutes at a time without feeling like I was going to faint. I suffered from back and leg pain and spasms. It was hard for me to grasp how my life could take such a disconcerting course after all my hard work. It left me feeling physically and emotionally challenged. In spite of this, I have been able to move through it with more resilience solely because I had put a wellness structure in place. You see, I had something to fall back on. So when my world began to unravel physically I had an improved ability to cope with the chronic pain, frustration and subsequent stress. I shudder to think of how I would have come through it if had not taken such good care of myself before it all started. That's not to say I don't have my down days, or that I'm not left frustrated and on the verge of tears from time to time.

Regardless of how much I tried to manage my health, my issues seemed to escalate out of my control. If you've ever studied the human body, you will know that it is a kinetic chain; that is everything is connected and when one element goes out of balance, either mechanically or chemically/hormonally, your body compensates and it will effect on other parts of your body. And that is exactly what happened.

Through a series of unfortunate accidents over the last few decades, my back has been continuously assaulted over the years. The degenerative process eventually caught up with me; consequently I am left with little more than the hairline remains of a disk in my lumbar spine between S1 and L5. The condition caused nerve impingement and intensely painful burning down the back of both of my legs to my feet. For nearly a year, every muscle in my lower legs was in spasm; my brain firing signals like a semi-automatic weapon.

My orthopedic physician, believed it to be a consequence of an accident and several past events came to mind; like the time I was in my early 20's and was intensely afraid of heights. I decided to face my fears head on and jump out of an airplane at 5000 feet. Certainly skydiving would remedy this silly fear and it was indeed a success, although I can't say it was worth the broken tailbone!

I was involved in several car accidents; hit by a guy on PCP, then by a cab driver who decided to play bumper cars with me. This last April I was rear ended by a woman in a cross-over SUV. Ironically, I was on my way to get a lower lumbar MRI in my small sports car. I saw the irony in this although it took me awhile to appreciate God's humor.

The last accident aggravated the existing pain to the point where I could not sit or stand more than a few minutes. I was becoming exhausted and my immune system was faltering. My mid-back was sore and burning due to the compensation from my low back. Bladder infections became frequent, and the yeast infections decided to party down under after each round of antibiotics. I was in a fog and was having great difficulty functioning and thinking clearly.

> *"Life is what happens in between our best-laid plans".*
> *Dr. Samir Sharma,*
> *Orthopaedic & Sports Medicine*

Eight days after getting rear ended, other unplanned life-events began vying for my attention. I noticed a lump in my left breast even though I had a clear mammogram just a few months prior. From the grating back pain, and stress of this new discovery, it created a string of migraines that had previously been eradicated.

Concurrently, my long time primary care physician, Dr. David Cahn, had conducted some lab work and detected my thyroid was at the lowest point of the normal range. Taking medication to balance the thyroid, within a week, I began experiencing heart palpitations and anxiety attacks.

At night, I would ask for my husband to hold my hand into the wee hours of the morning. With each tick of the clock, I felt like my life would implode. Wondering whether I would awake in the morning I left the TV on until I could hold my eyes open no longer.

After a couple of weeks, my anxiety continued to worsen in spite of my best efforts to "control" it. I would feel my heart rate slow, then race; my arm was numb, I had a crushing headache and tightness in my chest. 9-1-1 was on speed dial and couriered by ambulance to the hospital. I thought for certain they would check me out, and release me in the evening, that everything would be okay. After several hours it became evident they would admit me.

In the ER, the triage nurse asked me a series of questions: "Do you smoke?" "Do you drink" "Do you exercise?" I was privately congratulating myself for doing everything I could that lead up to this point in my life, to make all the choices I felt were in my best interest, for my health. In spite of my fear of having a heart issue, I felt reassured at least my lifestyle was not the cause of my potential demise.

Unable to sleep due to all the commotion throughout the night and hooked up to a portable heart monitor, I paced the sterile, darkened halls. In my fifties, I was clearly decades younger than all the ailing patients in the cardiac ward. Even though my landing here was caused by medication, as I later learned, it was frightening to see the consequences of either not taking care of oneself or having hereditary or age-related issues. The ward was full of frail elderly people, most unable to grace the halls at night as I was and confined to their beds due to stroke, heart attack and other serious issues. One emaciated woman in a neck brace was perched on the edge of her bed, simply staring. I could feel her isolation and loneliness knowing her time to move on was near.

After an exhausting and intensive battery of tests, I learned that I was hypersensitive to the thyroid medication –which I stopped abruptly—and that my heart was strong. Their conclusion allayed my fears and I could now move on to discover what was causing some of my other symptoms. The physician on staff suspected acid reflux due to a spasm I was feeling in my neck near my carotid artery. I had been taking anti-inflammatory medication for my back pain which I learned later created the reflux. This in turn caused my esophagus to spasm in my neck, limiting blood flow to my brain. Anxiety and an increased heart rate—caused by the thyroid medication—exacerbated the spasms. Only this last June, I was capable of walking about three minutes before nearly passing out; I felt as though my heart was pumping sludge through my veins.

Having the foresight to understand it was imperative to advocate for myself through the myriad of medical appointments, lab work, x-rays, medications and a multitude of specialists, I started taking detailed notes at the onset. I remember very little of the first half of the year so relied on these notes to make sense of the chaos. It was the tool I needed to provide information to my primary care physician as well as a hormone specialist, so they in turn could establish the connection between the thyroid medication related to my anxiety and racing heart, and the acid reflux. Discontinuing the prescription and OTC medications was what I needed to help recover.

For due diligence sake, I was curious what was happening with my reproductive hormones and sought out a highly recommended specialist, Dr. Margaret Mahoney. I assumed I was entering a peri-menopause phase as I am certainly of that age and I wanted to learn if any of my symptoms were due to hormonal imbalances. Dr. Mahoney was the consummate professional and was so thorough and thoughtful. After nearly two hours of discussion she helped me sort through my previous tests, procedures, medications and lab results. Her mind is sharp and her intuition well-tuned. She conducted two sets of lab tests, spaced three weeks apart to gage fluctuations in my estrogen, progesterone and testosterone. I was completely floored when she told me I have staved off menopause, that my ovaries were "robust" and functioning perfectly. I asked her what she could specifically attribute to this outcome and it all came down to my fitness level.

After this arduous year, I am appreciative I did all I could to prevent worse conditions and recovery quickly. Although my earlier accidents have left me with nothing more than a hairline remnant of a lower lumbar disk, I have been able to reduce my back pain through core training and some days I feel pain free. The writing of this book, incidentally, required a 30 minute "sit-stand-ice" cycle to manage the back pain. I am a work in progress and willing to do the work to stay well. I've have had a string of clear PAPs (do the happy-feet dance with me), and my migraines are so infrequent I am surprised when I get one. I am completely off my medications, am stronger, healthier, and happier. Each week provides encouraging improvement, and with each phase of my life that I encounter I feel better prepared to meet the next challenge.

Essentially, we never really "make it" to the end of some journey where we have met our wellness goals and we're done. We are a constant work in progress, requiring ongoing monitoring and adjustments as our lives unfold. Inevitably, we encounter stressors, injury, trauma or crisis, and need to self-evaluate and consider if our regimen needs modification. It is with this in mind as I look forward to monitoring my own health issues with an open mind and positive attitude.

This is actually the BEST time to get it into gear if you haven't yet. Get those hormones in check, boost your metabolism, energize your life, and live on the edge of your comfort zone. It's NEVER too late to change. At over 50, I have proven to myself that anything is possible. Thanks for allowing me to share my story with you.

CHAPTER 3

LIFESTYLE CHANGES FOR LIFE!

"If we don't change the direction we're going, we're likely to end up where we're headed."

~Ancient Chinese Proverb

Ultimately, we can't do the same thing we always do and expect a different outcome. Is it realistic to think that we can improve our health or well-being if we continue to eat the same unhealthy foods, not work out or exercise and continue to abuse our bodies?

If you don't feel as good as you would like, or your body isn't ultimately the way you want it to be right now, then something isn't working for you, and eating habits are not what they should be. If that's the case, it's time for a change. If you are not willing to be open-minded and make the changes necessary, then your body will never change—at least not for the better.

What is a Lifestyle Change?

"Good choices add up to habit, habit becomes instilled healthy behavior, and the behavior becomes your lifestyle, and even your preference."

~ Toni Julian

When we think of lifestyle changes terms like "change of life" and "hot flash" may come to mind, but I assure you that's not what I'm referring to; it is incorporating healthy eating and fitness choices as a part of our lifestyle to improve our health, well-being and quality of life and most importantly ensuring that it is **sustainable for the rest of our life**.

Sustainable lifestyle changes are choices we make on an hourly basis that we incorporate as part of our daily living. We start with one small change—one change only—and implement it once. It's about making the best choice you can, given the situation you are in at the time.

With that said, transformation of your body and health comes down to common sense, making good choices, a pinch of discipline and my favorite character trait: perseverance.

One of my favorite American icons once said, "You can have everything you want in life, just not always at the same time." I am going by memory so Oprah's quote may not be verbatim but I believe the gist is accurate and has resonated with me for decades. I can have what I want if willing to persevere; to disregard immediate gratification for a greater goal. It took me seven years to put myself through college while working full time, forfeiting a social life. I eventually earned my degree, but I had to sacrifice to attain my goal. The same goes with healthy lifestyle changes, they need to be regarded as a journey that will last a lifetime. A lean toned body and gorging on cheesecake every night are mutually exclusive.

When embarking on incrementally changing your habits, you need to cut yourself some slack and not be critical when you make less than optimal choices. This program is not a pass/fail eating plan. What you do need to do is make the best choice given your set of circumstances at that time, listen to feedback from your body, and when doing so, will develop healthier eating habits, that will in turn improve your metabolism and ensure sustainable results.

Where some people go off track is in thinking they have to revamp their entire lives overnight. And that's just not realistic. You think "I'm going to eat 1000 calories a day, plus get up at 5am for a run, then I'll hit the gym on the way home every night." The concern is that while it's a commendable commitment and initial effort, this really isn't a sustainable program because you will be hungry and sleep deprived. Your hormones will not function properly and will be driven to cravings and self-medicating through sugary, fatty foods and alcohol or caffeine. Unless changes are incorporated in a more incremental way, your life will go out of balance. Other priorities will begin to pull at your new routine, and you will likely go off track. Once off track, you may feel you failed and are hesitant to do anything new. Your old programming kicks in and reminds you that nothing you can do will work and that's simply just not true.

If you were to ask me, "was it easy?" regarding my own personal journey to a healthy lifestyle I would tell you that it's not hard if you start with one thing—and one thing only—and go from there. It becomes easier—then because you start to feel better very quickly, it motivates you to make more changes, which makes you feel even better. It's a highly motivating UPWARD spiral!

But you don't have the discipline you say? You only need a little bit of discipline when you are making small, incremental changes. And any shift in the right direction is progress.

Using common sense, getting back to basics, and being open to new ideas and willingness to do the work by INCREMENTALLY changing our current habits that we may not even realize are self-defeating—will take you a long way on your journey to regaining the vitality you so deserve.

REMEMBER: Lifestyle changes are about slowly changing your "old ways" in exchange for new healthier ones.

Take the Lifestyle Assessment

Check the most accurate response for each category. The top box is worth one point, the middle worth two points and the bottom box is worth three points.

1. Breakfast
   - ☐ Rarely or never
   - ☐ Most days of the week
   - ☐ Every morning

2. Eating Frequency
   - ☐ Often skip meals and may go for 5 to 6 hours without eating
   - ☐ 3 squares a day
   - ☐ Small meals every 3 to 4 hours

3. Food Quality
   - ☐ I eat mostly processed/refined foods and junk foods (microwave dinners, fast food)
   - ☐ I eat refined foods (pretzels, crackers, alcohol) along with relatively healthy food
   - ☐ I mostly eat fruits, vegetables, whole grains and lean proteins

4. Whole Grains
   - ☐ I typically eat white, starchy foods such as white rice, white bread
   - ☐ I try to limit "white processed foods" and make whole grains at least half of my intake
   - ☐ I buy and eat only 100% whole grain products

5. Food Preparation
   - ☐ I eat fried foods and foods prepared with heavy sauces and creams
   - ☐ I eat somewhere in between 1 and 3
   - ☐ I typically eat my foods either broiled, lightly stir-fried or raw

6. Eating Out
   - ☐ I eat out at restaurants for most of meals during the day
   - ☐ I eat out 2-3 times per week
   - ☐ I eat out only occasionally

7. Emotional Eating
   - ☐ I eat when I'm not hungry
   - ☐ I eat when I'm sad, mad, frustrated or bored
   - ☐ I eat when my body tells me to eat

8. Regularity
   - ☐ I have constipation problems and may go more than a few days at a time
   - ☐ I have bowl movements every other day
   - ☐ I have bowl movements once or twice every day

9. Bowel Consistency
   - ☐ Soft with a foul odor (or greasy)
   - ☐ Hard and dry (or pellet-like)
   - ☐ Medium-brown with consistency like peanut butter

10. Cardio Respiratory Exercise (prolonged elevated heart rate)
    - ☐ I'm very sedentary and do not do cardio (no, vacuuming doesn't count)
    - ☐ I do cardio exercise about three times each week
    - ☐ I walk, run, hike or do equivalent cardio exercises at least 30 minutes daily

11. Resistance Exercise and Core Training (using weights or your own body weight)
    - ☐ I do not do weight-bearing exercises or core work
    - ☐ I do weight-bearing exercises and core work occasionally
    - ☐ I do weight-bearing exercises and core work at least three days each week

12. Smoking
    - ☐ I smoke, either daily or "socially"
    - ☐ I quit smoking
    - ☐ I do not smoke

13. Alcohol Consumption
    - ☐ I have two to three drinks each day
    - ☐ I have two to three drinks each week
    - ☐ I do not drink

14. Water Consumption
    - ☐ I drink mostly sodas, coffee or wine
    - ☐ I drink at least 4 glasses of water daily (32 fl. oz.)

    ☐ I drink at least 8 glasses of water daily (64 fl. oz.)

15. Caffeine Intake
    ☐ I consume POWER drinks loaded with caffeine
    ☐ I consume caffeinated coffee or soda on a daily basis
    ☐ I do not consume caffeinated, or sweet (including diet) beverages

16. Sleep Hygiene
    ☐ I awake tired in the morning and know I'm not getting enough sleep
    ☐ My sleep is usually disrupted but feel rested most days
    ☐ I go to bed and rise at the same time each day and feel fresh in the morning

17. Medications
    ☐ I take 10 or more prescriptions or OTC medications on a daily basis
    ☐ I take several prescriptions or OTC medications daily
    ☐ I rarely, if ever, take prescription or OTC medications

Where are you on the lifestyle scale? Total your points and see the chart below.

48-51   You have developed exceptional lifestyle habits, stay on track!
37-47   Your lifestyle habits may need to be modified to reduce your health risk.
18-36   You're in need of a lifestyle makeover and may be in a high risk health category. See your doctor, get your blood work tested, and read on to optimize your lifestyle!

Where Should I Start?

The type of changes you make depends on where you are starting and where you want to be. For some we simply want to feel better, improve our energy, reduce the risk of illness and injury, or develop strength. To others we have weight issues and need to shed pounds to live in an optimally healthy range. Beyond that, we may have obesity issues and are at risk or suffering from diabetes, hypertension or heart disease. Lay on yet another layer of complexity for those with food allergies, sensitivities, or food related diseases such as Celiac.

Sustainable Lifestyle Change Examples

When making sustainable changes we can start anywhere. You will learn from your food journaling (as you will read in Chapter 15) which areas you may need to make some adjustments. Here are some examples of lifestyle changes and keep in mind some of these are transitional habits as starting places as you work toward your optimal lifestyle.

- ✓ Improving the quality of the foods you eat, and cut a few calories while you're at it, by limiting the number of times dining out at restaurants. Limit your excursions to one per week and view it as something special.
- ✓ Switch from the "white" processed flours to 100 percent whole wheat that includes bread, rice and pasta.
- ✓ Cut empty calories. Instead of drinking two glasses of wine every night, reduce it to one, saving nearly 1000 calories a week in the process. Then limit it to an occasional glass of wine once or twice each week. You may surprise yourself and not even miss it.
- ✓ Start packing your lunch for work. You pack your kids lunches, right? Offer yourself the same consideration!
- ✓ Step up your fitness game and instead of going to lunch at work with the team you lace up your walking shoes and hit the trail for 30 minutes each day. You've now just expended hundreds of extra calories in that given week while saving thousands of calories by packing your own healthy food.
- ✓ When you open the refrigerator for a snack, and you have many choices available to you ask yourself "is this a good choice, or is there a better one?" Remove yourself from the equation. Instead of what tastes good think "what is best for me?" Is it the left over chow mien or this yogurt with berries?
- ✓ Replace your evening dessert with Good Earth Original tea to cut the sweet craving, or a green apple and 10 almonds.

✓ Switch from caffeinated to decaffeinated coffee. Use half of each to transition until it's purely decaffeinated.

✓ Transition from drinking sugary sodas to diet beverages, then to sparkling water with a splash of fruit juice (like cranberry), then to water with a squirt of lemon, lime, cucumber or mint for a refreshing drink.

✓ Cut down on the fat you use when cooking. Use nonstick cooking spray (just enough to moisten the pan) instead of pats of butter or pouring oils into the pan for frying.

✓ Switch from ground beef to ground turkey, then lean ground turkey.

✓ Start using a measuring cup and scale at the table so you can start becoming aware of portion sizes.

✓ Get to bed 30 minutes earlier than usual, and increase that time until you feel refreshed in the morning and are getting the optimal amount of sleep.

✓ Stop buttering your toast

This last checkpoint may sound insignificant but anything you do adds up over time. And yes, it may be as simple as eating your toast dry instead of a 100 calorie pat of butter every day. By changing this one little habit, you will lose a pound of fat in three weeks. Back in college I was a "healthy" size 11. I attributed this mostly to my desire for sweets, eating low quality foods and an increasingly sedentary lifestyle. While obsessed with gymnastics in high school, I had no fitness replacement. I worked full time and studied when I wasn't working. Very quickly, I found myself looking more "corn-fed" than healthy. I was motivated to start making lifestyle changes and found that if I didn't butter my bread, I gradually started to lean down. Over the next few years I was back to my size 6 jeans, without dieting.

What a lifestyle change is not: is some magic diet plan or instantaneous solution to weight loss or health issues. As I mentioned before, the objective of any lifestyle change is that it is sustainable.

CHAPTER 4

WHY DIETS DON'T WORK

"I highly recommend worrying. It is much more effective than dieting."
~William Powell

Essentially every bite of food that goes into your mouth is considered your "diet." Popular food diets however are different in the way they have a set program that encourages you to buy their food or is based on deprivation and depletion of nutrients and your lean mass. Many of these fad "diets" are not sustainable because they are restrictive and we end up feeling deprived, hungry, fatigued and cranky. We can only adhere to them for so long before we go back to our old ways.

In our world of instant results, our expectations increasingly lean toward a quick fix, and we'll believe in almost any new diet or gimmick that comes our way. Desperate, we invest our hopes and beliefs in a diet plan, supplement, or herbal remedy we are told will be the solution to all our problems. Many claims are utterly ridiculous but we hold onto the hope that maybe this one will be "it"!

I am not an advocate of any popular "diet program". They are misleading at best. Certainly you can go on a high protein/low carbohydrate diet or a cabbage soup or cookie diet and lose weight initially, but the overwhelming majority of the dieters will gain all their weight back and then some. Yes, you may know someone who was successful at keeping it off for years, but if you surveyed everyone you knew you'd find 95 people out of 100 went on "diets" and gained their weight back, and then some, many times over.

The absolutely worst part about diets is how they make people feel. This morning I met a nice 40-something woman at the gym locker room and she told me she could not remember which locker was hers and that she has trouble mentally functioning after a workout, so of course I asked her how she was eating. She proceeded to tell me she is on a popular diet program (I'll exclude the name) and she just felt horrible. She had no energy, her mind was in a fog and I was concerned. I told her the problem with that is it's just not sustainable. She is clearly not getting enough carbohydrates otherwise she would be able to think clearly. Her blood sugar was so low, leaving her feeling depleted. What she didn't know is that her body was now resorting to tearing down the muscle to use as fuel. This is the story with so many people I encounter. They focus on scale weight only and really need to learn how their body functions in order to not only find results, but make it work with their life in the process.

Imagine cutting out all carbohydrates and trying to sustain popular high protein diets . . . it would throw us into withdrawal. We need those complex carbohydrates to fuel our brain and our body. In preparation for a Figure Competition I reduced my carbohydrates in the week before the "big day." I craved them so desperately; like a drug, I was texting my trainer to find out where I could find a Carbohydrates Anonymous meeting for support. If we deprive ourselves, we are setting ourselves up for failure. And high protein diets are hard not only hard on our liver but for every gram of protein we eat above our basic tissue maintenance requirements, we lose 1 to 1.5 grams of Calcium right along with it. High protein diets are also associated with an increased saturated fat intake and reduced fiber intake, both increasing the risk for some types of cancer as well as heart disease.

What about a cookie diet? You eat a cookie for every meal (which is loaded with unhealthy sugars, fats and white flour) then eat a balanced dinner, plus include a solid workout each day. Anyone would lose weight if they ate any food item at 150 calories (say, half a Snickers bar) for each meal then ate a "reasonable" dinner, and added exercise. But the question is what kind of weight and what are you doing to your body as a result of this yo-yo approach? There's nothing special or healthy about these fad diets on the market so to these folks I say "BITE ME!" Good common sense should always prevail.

We all know someone who is a "yo-yo" dieter. They are caught in a vicious cycle of depriving themselves, losing weight, eating normally, gaining the weight back—and then some—and starting the dieting process all over again. Over time, their metabolism is reduced, and often they are much larger as an end result than if they didn't diet at all.

If your goal is weight loss, it is not as straightforward as it seems. What truly works may be counterintuitive to what we think we know because of all the misinformation we receive. Some weight loss experts, even doctors or nutritionists, prescribe an 800 calorie per day diet, some primarily consisting of supplements. Concept: reduce calories, lose weight.

If we cut calories too severely, we may be consuming inadequate protein and calories; our blood sugar drops. Deprivation diets contribute to a loss of lean muscle mass, which in turn lowers metabolism. If we're not giving our muscles the nutrients required for maintenance our body begins burning the glucose in the muscle for fuel. In turn, we lose muscle mass, and our metabolism drops because muscle requires more calories to sustain it per pound than body fat. In other words, eat less than 300 calories under your BMR (Basil Metabolism Rate), which is how many calories your body requires to function metabolically without movement or exercise, and your muscles become your body's fuel.

CHAPTER 5

RETRAINING YOUR METABOLISM

In the previous chapter we discussed how you can destroy your metabolism. Now let's talk about how to build it up. We can accomplish this by first understanding how your body works metabolically.

Our bodies function in a miraculous way. Simplistically, sleep heals the body, quality (nutritious) food and resistance training builds the muscle, and exercise burns the fat. Having all these elements in balance will put your body in homeostasis.

Homeostasis is keeping your body balanced ensuring your blood sugar (glucose) levels are stable at all times. When your blood sugar is stable, within 80-120 mg/dl, our bodies release fatty acids to be burned. Too few calories and we are hungry, experience cravings and fatigue. Too many calories and we store fat and have decreased energy for exercise and experience blood sugar lows. In order to accomplish this balance we must maintain a healthy blood sugar level so our bodies will work efficiently.

Feed yourself adequate calories, eat frequently, and at a slight deficit (burn about 300-500 calories more per day than you eat) you can re-train your body to understand that it can let go of the fat, there is no need to stubbornly store it as fuel in preparation for the next famine. Our bodies are programmed to crave fat, sugar and salt as a way to ensure survival. Lose it slowly as a lifestyle change and you will keep it off.

NewsBite: Which weighs more, a pound of muscle or a pound of fat?
You got it, they weigh the same! But did you know that fat takes up three times the amount of volume? And, a pound of fat burns only a couple of calories each day, whereas a pound of muscle burns between 30-50 calories. Boost your metabolism by increasing your lean muscle mass. If you gained six pounds of muscle, you may need as much as an extra 300 calories per day just to maintain it.

The solution is BALANCE. Eat a little bit of everything in each meal: lean protein, complex carbohydrates and healthy, unsaturated fats in moderation. You will not feel deprived or hungry if you approach your eating habits this way. It's not about being perfect, or eating perfectly, but about making the best possible choice you can, given your set of circumstances. Your choices add up to behavior, that behavior becomes habit; the habit is now your lifestyle and perhaps even your preference.

1. **Eat enough calories at each meal**. Women typically need 250-300 calories per meal, while men need around 400.
2. **Eat frequent meals:** Eating small meals every 3-4 hours will regulate your blood sugar and keep you in a fat burning mode. Skip meals and your glucose levels will plummet initiating a chain reaction of hormones causing your body to hold onto the fat. Your goal: 5-6 small meals daily.
3. **Eat the proper balance:** Consume lean protein, complex carbohydrates and healthy fats to keep you satiated, and keep your body in homeostasis (blood sugar balance)
4. **Eat breakfast:** It will boost your metabolism for the rest of the day
5. **Incorporate resistance training**. Weight training will not only build muscle but help keep your skeletal structure strong

as well. More muscle means a higher metabolism as energy is burned in the muscle.

6. **Listen to feedback from your body:** if you have had a high caloric expenditure day and are feeling extra hungry, add another meal to your day, not more calories to your existing meals.

7. **Exercise a minimum 30 minutes every day** –and keep it productive. Focus on hill climbing, or a treadmill walk at an incline. Now that your body is in balance through eating healthy, it's time to burn the fat!

CHAPTER 6

BLOOD SUGAR—A DELICATE BALANCE

We all understand the need for balance in our lives; we practice it every day. We juggle all the elements; work, family and friends, exercise, nutrition and sleep. The focus is external, in other words, the activities in our life taking place on the outside.

Our body has a balance on the inside as well and the key to our wellness lies in our ability to keep our bodies in homeostasis, a physiological balance of our internal systems. Our organs all have specific functions, taking stewardship of these systems—especially our endocrine system—releasing hormones for metabolism and blood glucose (sugar) regulation.

As I've mentioned before, our nutrition—what we eat—has the most significant impact on how we look and feel, because of its contribution to homeostasis. When I talk with my clients, their main goal is typically to feel better; the secondary goal is focused on weight loss. They tend to "feel better" when their blood sugar is in balance, not too low (hypoglycemia) and not too high (hyperglycemia) but within an appropriate range. According to the National Diabetes Information Clearinghouse, the optimal range for non-diabetic people are 70-99 mg/dl upon waking, and 70-140 mg/dl after meals.[1]

---

1   American Diabetes Association, Standards of medical Care in diabetes—2008

Incorrect eating habits contribute to an upset in a delicate homeostatic balance. As a consequence, we not only suffer the effects of blood sugar highs and lows, but the abuse of this balance tends to set us up to store fat when our glucose levels are high and burn muscle as fuel when it's too low.

Low blood sugar is defined as an inadequate supply of glucose to the brain. Symptoms include hunger, shakiness, nervousness, sweating, dizziness or light-headedness, sleepiness, confusion, difficulty speaking, anxiety and weakness. Some effects many even include low blood sugar episode in your sleep, causing headaches upon awaking and nightmares.[2]

A side note regarding migraines: I had experienced occasional nightmares and would wake with a crushing migraine. It was only after conducting research on low blood sugar did I realize there was a direct correlation in between the two, at least in my world. I knew low blood sugar was one of my many triggers when it came to migraines; what I didn't realize is that one could suffer its effects during sleep. Anxiety is another personal migraine trigger, so I always questioned whether it was the anxiety from the nightmare that triggered the migraine, or did the migraine trigger the nightmare? I mention this as food for thought so you can delve into finding your triggers if you are in fact a migraine suffer as I am. I found low blood sugar was a constant variable during all my migraine episodes.

NewsBite: A fascinating bit of information, according to the National Institute of Health, alcohol can cause hypoglycemia (low blood sugar) even a few days after consumption. This delay creates greater difficulty in trying to correlate the effects of your diet to headaches, or migraines, which makes journaling even more important and gives you a tool to resolve the issue.

---

2   National Diabetes Information Clearinghouse (NDIC) Hypoglycemia NIH Publication No. 09-926 October 2008 (website article

So what causes our blood sugar to rise too quickly? Eating too many overly processed carbohydrate foods, such as white rice, on an empty stomach without combining it with protein and healthy fat, and eating too many calories at one meal, will contribute to rise in blood glucose (sugar) level and ultimate fat storage.

Waiting too long between meals—or worse yet—skipping a meal, causes blood sugar to drop, forcing the body to metabolize lean muscle for energy. Lose muscle and the body requires fewer calories each day to support the muscle, meaning you have to eat slightly less as your metabolism drops. Although the exact number is controversial, the majority of sources agree that for every pound of muscle lost, you will need to reduce calories by around 25-30 every day just to break even.

How does this work on a hormonal level? Insulin, a hormone produced by the pancreas, is released with a mission to drive the high levels of glucose into your fat cells for storage. Another hormone, glucagon, counterbalances the insulin and strives to increase blood sugar levels when they fall too low. If we continue to allow our blood sugar to spike and plummet, eventually our ability to produce insulin and/or glucagon may be impacted and could potentially result in pre-diabetes and Diabetes Type II.

The good news . . . when your blood sugar is stable, somewhere within 80-120 mg/dl; our bodies release fatty acids to be burned. Too few calories and we are hungry, experience cravings and fatigue. Too many calories and we store fat and have decreased energy for exercise and experience blood sugar lows. In order to accomplish this balance we must maintain a healthy blood sugar level so our bodies will work efficiently.

Stabilize your blood sugar level by eating the right combination of the three types of foods—lean protein, complex carbohydrates (no white, processed carbs!) and healthy fats—and eating small meals throughout the day—will help to keep these levels regulated.

Imagine your blood glucose level cruising along on a track of steep climbs and stressful plummets. A typical diet for many—identified as "Mean Eating Routine" and is actually a snapshot of a typical day for me a few years ago—shows how we skip breakfast and a morning snack, perhaps subsisting on coffee until we overindulge at lunch and over consume calories, the extra calories being stored as fat. Because we have eaten such an overly substantial lunch, we don't feel the need for an afternoon snack, but we're ravenous again by dinner and consume the greatest amount of calories for that meal. Overall, our bodies feel depleted due to lack of quality food, and carbohydrate cravings occur after dinner. These of course are simple sugars, spike our glucose levels and result in further fat storage.

Below two scenarios are presented to illustrate how blood sugar spikes throw your body into fat storing mode, and how low blood sugar will cause your body to resort to tearing down your muscles for fuel.

Mean Eating Routine

Breakfast:	Coffee
Snack:	None
Lunch:	Lean Cuisine, Diet Soda
	(Low in nutrients and calories, high in sodium)
Snack:	None
Dinner:	Lasagna, sourdough bread, salad with ranch dressing, 2 glasses red wine
Evening Snack:	Brandy, chips and chocolate

Toni's New Lean Eating Routine:

Breakfast:	French Toast (whole wheat w/egg whites) and Fruit
Morning Snack:	Edamame and Bran Muffin
Lunch:	Turkey Bean Soup, Brown Rice and Quinoa, Steamed or Sautéed Veggies
Afternoon Snack:	Cottage Cheese, Fruit, Raw Almonds
Dinner:	Grilled Salmon, Mixed Baby Greens, Yummy Yam Fries, 4 oz. Red Wine
Evening Snack:	Hummus, Red Pepper Strips and Walnuts

Notice the differences in the two meal plans: The first shows a skipped breakfast, long periods of time between meals resulting in low blood sugar, the majority of the calories hitting at bedtime, way too much alcohol resulting in a calorie overload, and highly processed, high glycemic foods contributing to blood sugar spikes and promotion of fat storage.

Next, look at how the new plan addresses all those incorrect eating behaviors. Every meal is perfectly balanced; combining a lean protein, a complex carbohydrate and a healthy fat. Notice the variety of nutrients, whole grains, inclusion of vegetables and fruits. Overall the quality of the food is much higher (A few ounces of red wine during dinner are considered healthy by many sources although you need to determine what is best for you). An evening snack should be eaten only if hungry.

Finally, check out the amount of food in both plans, the new plan I am eating six meals a day and consuming a large volume of food. The beauty is because the foods are whole, high quality and combined properly, I'm satiated at every meal and eating far fewer calories overall.

The chart below symbolizes the two scenarios. Regulated blood sugar falls between the ideal range of 80 mg/dl and 120 mg/dl.

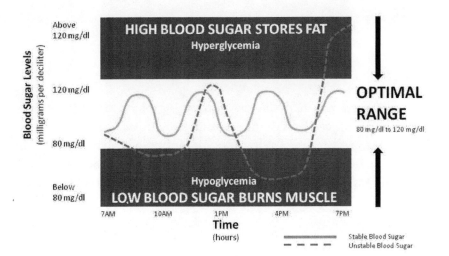

Lowering Your Glycemic Load

Most of us are familiar with the Glycemic Index (GI); it's based on how quickly carbohydrates break down and effect blood sugar levels.

In simplified terms, the Glycemic Index runs on a relative scale of one to over 100—with 100 being the relative rating for the measurement for glucose; processed and refined foods and simple sugars are broken down more quickly causing insulin to be released and are found on the high end, whereas complex carbohydrates, such as grains, and most fruits and vegetables are more difficult to break down and are at the lower end of the Glycemic Index. Some examples from the Glycemic Index Foundation rank (glucose) sugar at 100, while an artichoke is only 15.[3]

Below are the general ranges:

High GI 70 and above	**Medium GI** 56-69	**Low GI** 0-55
Baked Potatoes	Whole Wheat Pasta	Fruits
White Bread	Whole Wheat Bread	Vegetables (Including Carrots)
White Rice	Sweet Potatoes	Beans
Processed Breakfast	Cereals	Nuts
Glucose (Sugar—All Forms)		
	Whole Grains(Quinoa, Brown Rice)	
	Yams	

However there are many factors to lowering blood sugar levels than simply looking at the GI index. And you must also factor in the reality that just because it is lower on the GI scale, it may not have the nutritional benefits of a food that is higher on the scale. So taking both nutrition and the index into account is the optimal way to make food choices. You can lower the overall effect of the meal—the Glycemic

---

3   Glycemic Index Foundation, The University of Sidney 2011

Load—first by understanding how your body processes foods, then through proper food choices.

When you eat, carbohydrates begin to be broken down in the mouth by enzymes in the saliva into simpler compounds. Proteins and fats begin this process in the stomach and absorption of nutrients takes place in the small intestine.

Important Tips:

- ✓ By eating 50% of calories from carbohydrates low on the Glycemic Index, that person can have the same calories and benefit from more stable blood sugar and insulin levels
- ✓ Combining a combination of carbohydrates, with lean proteins and healthy fats, slows the carbohydrate breakdown and glucose absorption
- ✓ Glycemic response (an individual response to the same food) will vary from person to person
- ✓ Consuming fewer calories overall, losing weight, and keeping carbohydrates to 50% of your diet have significant impact on blood glucose levels
- ✓ Blood glucose levels are affected by previous meals
- ✓ A small amount of alcohol just before a meal can actually lower the GI of the meal by 15% (Alcohol has calories, but not carbohydrates)

If you want to eat a high Glycemic food, such as chocolate for example, and want to minimize a blood sugar spike, resulting in a low blood sugar drop later, first eat some lean protein and a healthy fat first. The protein and fat will slow the digestion of the high GI food, decreasing the overall load and helping to minimize an insulin spike. If you are Diabetic though, speak to your doctor about your specific needs.

Good Sleep Hygiene

Getting enough sleep is your foundation for a healthy lifestyle. Lack of sleep raises cortisol levels, increasing your blood pressure, stress and blood sugar levels. Cortisol levels increase your appetite; sugar cravings lead to consumption of empty calories, both contributing to weight gain. How much sleep should you get? We are all genetically different and some people do well on five or six hours, while others need more. If you have enough sleep, you should wake feeling refreshed, not exhausted.

Tips for a good night's sleep

- ✓ Schedule the correct number of hours for sleep and wake at the same time
- ✓ Avoid naps, unless there are at a consistent time every day
- ✓ Avoid excessive time in bed
- ✓ Clear your brain, journal your thoughts, or list items on your mind for the next day
- ✓ Expose yourself to bright light when awake, and a dark environment at night
- ✓ Avoid nicotine, caffeine, alcohol and simple carbohydrates, especially late in the day
- ✓ Exercise regularly and early in the morning
- ✓ Eat a light snack before bedtime if hungry, lean protein is best
- ✓ Relax! Stretch or read before bed
- ✓ If noise is a problem, invest in some earplugs; try out several types to see which best suit you

In a perfect world we would all go to sleep and wake at the same time each day, but sometimes situations or events undermine our ability to do this. Perhaps you have business travel, are stressed about a relationship or your baby has an ear-infection, and your sleep is interrupted. You need to be able to manage these sleep deficits immediately rather than let them pile up to the end of the week and crash.

So what should you do if you have a poor night's sleep? Get back on track immediately. Let's say you stayed up until midnight reading an engrossing book that you just "could not put down!" and you had only five hours of sleep but you needed eight leaving you with a three-hour deficit. Here's a tool you can implement right away.

Rather than nap, likely throwing off your sleep cycle set a new schedule to make up the specific three-hour deficit. If you typically wake at 7am every day, and you need eight hours of sleep, you would normally need to be asleep by 11pm. Go to bed one hour earlier—at 10pm. Repeat this for three consecutive nights, being sure to wake at the same time each day. You will feel better each day, and energized by the third day. And if you are eating right, you will feel ready to take on the world.

CHAPTER 7

YOUR POSITIVE ATTITUDE
WILL SET YOU FREE!

"The greatest discovery of all time is that a person can change his future by merely changing his attitude."

-Oprah Winfrey

Ever meet an enormously positive person and watch how others are drawn to them? They look at the world with an "I CAN" attitude and their optimism is contagious. They believe in miracles, they believe in change. They do not declare defeat before embarking on a new journey with self-doubt and negative talk. These people give you energy, while negativity, quite bluntly, will suck the life out of you.

I met one of these truly inspirational people, Margaret Hyde, about ten years ago on a walk through our hilly neighborhood paths. Through a brief conversation with her I had learned she had a hip replacement and I simply admired her persevering attitude. Now, at 80 years old, through one of our chance and brief encounters along the very same path, she shared with me that she had been going through a difficult year and it was the first time she had been on the trail in months. She mentioned her husband was ill and my heart went out to her. I asked her to tell me what keeps her going. As she opened her arms as if to embrace the universe she said "I'm intoxicated with life!" And I said that's how I feel too! Margaret is one of those people who I would be fortunate enough to emulate. Her spirit is bright and strong, her attitude positive, and her heart simply sings in spite of it all. We can all learn a little something from her.

If you find yourself doubtful of your ability to change your lifestyle, I would challenge you to shift your thinking just a bit and you'll see how successful you will be. If you don't think you can do something, you will be certain to live up to that low expectation. Free yourself of any negative thinking. If your catch yourself thinking an undermining thought, re-state that thought in a positive way. If you think, "Oh why should I bother?" when it comes to eating well, think again. "I recognize taking care of me takes time, and I'm worth the investment." Self-correct your thoughts as you go along.

Set realistic, attainable expectations of yourself. If you are recovering from an injury, as I am, I know I need to modify my thinking and be appreciative for the things I can do, rather than focus on what I can't. I can't run, but I CAN hike the hill, I CAN ride my bike.

Accomplished milestones will fuel your self-esteem, making you feel good about what you are doing. As my clients perform their "plank" exercise some hit the 3 minute mark and they are justifiably proud when they initially could hold for only 15 to 30 seconds. Every additional 15 seconds is an accomplished milestone to be recognized.

When people ask you "How are you?" always say, "I'm well, thank you!" and avoid the lengthy bemoaning and accounting of every ache and pain. If you believe you are well in your mind, you will feel better than thinking and dwelling on the things that make you not well.

When you go on a walk, to the gym, or your favorite class, wear more fitted exercise clothes, not boxy, oversized T-shirts and sweats. You will feel better not hiding behind clothes that make your booty look like a sack of potatoes. If there is a mirror where you work out you will see your muscles flex and will be more encouraged if you have a visual. It will also help you establish a neuromuscular connection, the way your brain communicates with a specific muscle, and you will become more efficient and get more out of your workout that way.

Even around the house or running an errand, put on a little make-up, a touch of mascara, some blush and lip gloss. If you feel pretty, you will feel better about yourself, be more approachable and have an improved outlook on your day.

Keep yourself surrounded by supportive, positive people. My mom once said people either make you feel small or make you feel big. Simple words but so very true. Keep company with people who lift you up when you need it. Be selective about who you chose to be in your inner circle. There are times when we all need encouragement. No one deserves to be belittled or dragged down. Allow the positive to fuel your soul. Freeing yourself from doubt and defeating self-talk is liberating . . . you just might be surprised at where your positive thinking will take you! Your new mantra: I'm intoxicated with life!

Your True Motivation

Anyone can lose weight; many of us have demonstrated that over and over again. The real questions are, how can you motivate yourself to want to make healthful changes, how can you keep it off and how do we decide to get back on course if we've strayed?

I believe there are two forms of motivational strategies that are useful; the first is short term motivation and the second is long term. In the short term, we need to recognize that we don't need an enormous amount of motivation if we make small, incremental changes that are manageable. Live with the changes for a while; become accustomed to them until they become habits. Remember, you don't need a lot of motivation if you are not depriving yourself.

Long term motivation comes from deep in the gut. And to get to the heart of your unique driving force; the honest, naked truth that will spur you on to your goal, you need to continue to ask yourself, "Why?"

The answer to your "why" will provide the deep motivation needed to ensure the changes you are making sustainable for life. If you find a meaningful reason to change toward a healthier lifestyle, it will give you a strong purpose to propel you to meet your goal. From time to time, everyone gets thrown off their game. So dig deep, and ask yourself "why" until you get to the underlying reason for wanting to make changes.

Here is a real-life example from a client who wished to remain anonymous:

"My goal is to lose 40 pounds within 12 months".

"Why?"
"Because I'll look better in my clothes"
Why do you want to look better in your clothes?
"So people will pay attention to me."
Why do you want people to pay attention to you?
"So I won't feel invisible."
Why don't you want to feel invisible?
"I want to feel important and my self-esteem is slipping."
Why is your esteem slipping?
"Because my husband doesn't think I am attractive anymore and won't have sex with me."

Deep motivation: So my husband will be intimate with me again.

Other potential motivators:

- ✓ So my daughter will be proud of me and not embarrassed around her friends
- ✓ So I will have the energy to play with my grandchildren
- ✓ So my athletic performance will improve and I'll be more competitive
- ✓ So I can minimize my chronic pain
- ✓ So I can enjoy outdoor activities with my family and not feel left out

Everyone's motivation will be different. Find out what yours is so you may keep focused on your goals and find the inner strength to fall back on. True motivation is powerful. Keep it in the forefront of your mind.

CHAPTER 8

ARM YOURSELF WITH ASSERTION SKILLS, A FORK AND AN ATTITUDE

"It is unbelievable that at age 50 I am worried about how other people are going to judge what I eat!"

~ Sue Lewis

Asserting your right to eat well and not being afraid to stand up to undermining influences will take you a long way in ensuring your success. So get prepared. Just say "BITE ME!" to Societal Expectations, Misinformation, Food Industry Deceptions and Fast Food InFATuation.

Societal Expectations

There are limitless social opportunities for indulging. We may have several birthdays, lunches, parties and gatherings each week and are in the position to eat clean or go with the flow. To eat healthy actually goes against the social grain and losing weight, or choosing to make healthy lifestyle choices, may make others feel uncomfortable. My belief is that they are witnessing you be your own advocate for change, and they know deep inside they should be doing the same. Their expectation is that you eat like they do, so they don't feel badly in comparison. Those closest to us are impacted the most, and they are the very people from whom we need the most support. However not all life partners are on the same path. It requires an understanding of this dynamic, along with a slightly indignant attitude, to persevere.

Let's face it; going against the grain is simply not easy. It's a bit like skydiving. I remember in my 20's a junior college buddy asked me if I'd like to go. I quickly said "sure" without really thinking it through. I was afraid of heights. I justified it by thinking that I should face my fears head on. The instructor at the skydiving school strapped a parachute pack on my back that weighed almost as much as me at the time; it was 75 pounds on my 115-pound frame. Up in the plane, I was white with fear as I scooted my booty toward the opening in the small plane. I swiveled my legs over the edge and it felt like a wild river at my feet. Bracing against the side of the opening, and barely able to keep them in place against the current, I threw myself out into the abyss, tumbling, tumbling until my shoot opened at the end of the taught static line. Suddenly, it was calm and smooth and although I was plummeting through the air, I felt no resistance to the wind because I was going with it, not against it. The feeling of striving to eat healthy against the current of those who don't had given me the same disoriented feeling in the beginning of my journey. It took a little time to become accustomed to the turbulence before it evened out.

Early on, I experienced an unexpected consequence of making changes is that as I modified my eating behaviors, I was no longer on the same page with family and friends. I would pick up subtle, and at times outright overt, comments about how boring I was that I wouldn't drink alcohol or eat crap at parties, that life is about having fun and how could I possibly feel it was worth it to give this up? After all, life is too short not to indulge. My reaction: Life will be short if I do. The implication is that eating healthy and making it delicious is mutually exclusive. The mindset is how can I possibly enjoy myself without over-indulging in unhealthy foods? How can we possibly have any fun in life if we are denying ourselves the very sustenance that makes this country great? And sick . . . and fat!

I feel a little like Carrie on Sex and the City, as I see the words across my computer appear letter by letter: "Can't I be the life of the party without the party being the death of me?" We're not on high school anymore, and I can have fun without getting hammered. Now whether or not other people think I am fun to be around when not drinking; that is really their issue, not mine. With confidence, I know I will be feeling great the next day, knowing they'll be up close and personal with the inside rim of their toilet bowl.

If you have food sensitivities as I do there is nothing fun about feeling sick all the time, about waking up with a migraine after only two glasses of wine or feeling hung over all day long after eating what I call the Super-Bowl party buffet. We've all been there, searching for a remnant of healthy food among the pizza, Buffalo wings and meatballs marinating in a fatty sauce.

At times we have to assert our right to eat well. It can be done in a way that is polite, or more overtly direct, depending upon how far we are pushed. When I first began clean-eating, my defense was to simply ignore it. In one instance, one of my friends made an ice cream sundae at a party and handed it to me, telling me to eat it. I was stupefied, how could consuming all this headache-inducing sugar possibly be in my best interest? It was well-intentioned, but also lacked understanding around my medical and personal needs. I laughed it off and left it on the counter to melt into oblivion. However I have to say it is gratifying when someone is simply pushy and I can come back with a polite smile and say, "Bite me!"

Just last year, I went to my sister's birthday and found myself at a restaurant amongst a great group of female family and friends, who, as the party progressed, it became evident that two separate groups were forming. We had the healthy-lifestyle minimally-drinking, clean-eating, "BITE ME!" fans, and then collecting at the other end of the table sat the martini-drinking, appetizer-ordering, pass-the-bread-basket-please group. Friction ensued to the point that some of the ladies began looking suspiciously at everyone's food choices and exchanging looks. It was like a group of Democrats on one end and Republicans on the other. Can't we live in a bi-partisan world without a food fight ensuing?

For a while I could not escape the criticism, even at home. Setting the dinner table, I always included a measuring cup and scale so I could learn portion control and serving sizes. Now I can estimate and don't use the scale anymore, but learning how much and what is in my foods is imperative in the beginning; although it definitely elicited some good-natured chiding from my family!

One of my clients, Heather, has been incredibly successful with asserting her right to eat well. She told me, "*It seems like the cleaner you eat, and the better you feed yourself with nutrients, society is so quick to judge, or make fun of you. You are really going against the normalcy that Americans today are being brought up knowing. I embraced this program, adopting clean eating and was very excited about it so shared it with my friends. This didn't sit well with everyone in my world. I was called out for being obsessed or going "over board." I thought to myself, there are worse things in life to be obsessed about, I took it as a compliment, and continued on with my journey. I had a specific altercation happen with someone very close to me, whom I talked with on regular basis and still do. I was speaking of my day, and all its encounters, and brought up something I had learned that day that related to health; and I was condemned for it. As if I was becoming a bore to talk with on the phone. Seems crazy to me now, but I had to sit back and ask myself who I was doing this for? And all fingers pointed back to me! I was worth it, and anything that is different isn't always accepted and understood at first. I choose at that point, with this person, that I would offer the information when asked and nothing more. I had to keep my healthy conversations with the people who were on this wave-length with me, and understood what I was after. It's a very neat concept that I will continue to capture and endure for the rest of my life regardless of what the grain says. I choose the path that is best suited for me, and the lifestyle I have adopted.*"

Lifestyle changes can be certain to test relationships, as Heather experienced. Another one of my client's wives (we'll call him Aeron) came to me a few months ago, very concerned about her husband. She said he looked drawn and his compulsion toward all this healthy eating was creating conflict in their marriage. She recognized there was some mild friction prior to his new lifestyle change, but that it made it worse. I clearly recognized the divide between them. He had lost a significant amount of weight—over 100 pounds—by following the guidelines in my book and improved his health immensely. Once sedentary, he was no longer limited in his activities, incorporating hiking, trips and adventures into his life. It was unlikely she was able to participate at his level; they were no longer on the same page. He ate only clean healthy foods and using his detail-oriented, technical talents, was fanatic about tracking them. It served him well in losing the weight and getting him to his goal of maintenance. But now she wanted it to end. He had essentially improved the quality of his life, while hers had not changed.

It's interesting how much support you get if you have blocked arteries and say you can't have saturated fats and avoid the beef ribs at the next barbeque. Everyone understands that. But if you want to be proactive and eat healthy it is more commonly met with confusion, because it is our nature to be more reactive, than proactive when it comes to our health. We will take our cars in for maintenance, have the oil changed, replace the brake pads and get a lube job. We get the term "prevention" when it comes to ensuring our car warranty remains in place. But guess what, we don't have a warranty on our lives. Why don't we get it? Would Aeron's wife have felt the same if he had a stroke before initiating his lifestyle change, instead of being proactive?

And how do you proactively solicit the health of a partner whose support you need? You've decided to venture on a journey toward better health, and you would like their support. You may be changing aspects about your life and you'd like to include him/her. Make it a part of their choice to be included or excluded. That's the operative word, choice. It is your choice to exercise, make good eating decisions, and get to bed at a reasonable hour. It is their choice, to participate in the process, or not. Some partners may not be supportive, and it may be overt and obvious, or they be more passive-aggressive about it and it may be more difficult for you to identify the behavior because while they "say" they are supportive, what they "do" is incongruous. I tend to go by people's actions instead of their words.

As you improve the quality of your life, start feeling amazing, and can enjoy yourself more thoroughly, those around you will either be with you, cheering you on, left behind possibly feeling threatened, or perhaps somewhere in between. You will be more successful if you have the support of loved ones and if you approach this together, and will be in a better position to help each other. However we cannot force this or control what other people do. If they want no part of this you can at least act as a role model, leading by example. Feeling and looking good can be contagious.

When it comes to making proactive, healthy choices, remember: this is YOUR life, and YOUR body, and your decisions should be based on supporting your health while knowing the people around you are not impacted in a negative way.

Now, armed with new knowledge, an understanding of how your body metabolizes food, and how to keep your body in homeostasis, you chose when to indulge and when to eat clean, it should be on your terms, not out of obligation or concern that you will go against the grain if you don't partake. To people who don't understand that refer them back to the title of this book. Just say, "BITE ME!" then be strong!

Misinformation

> "Even if we give parents all the information they need and we improve school meals and build brand new supermarkets on every corner, none of that matters if when families step into a restaurant, they can't make a healthy choice."
>
> ~ Michelle Obama

What to believe. There is so much information available—online, in advertising, and product labeling creating misconceptions as far as what is healthy. We are bombarded by companies with self-serving agendas, told we are "treating ourselves" when the food is actually destructive. And product labeling can be outright deceptive. We are tricked into believing food products are either healthier for us or have better quality ingredients by the way they spin their packaging claims.

Many processed or packaged foods tout, "0 Trans Fat," or say, "natural," "organic," or "gluten-free," but are loaded with artery clogging saturated fat, are explicitly designed to mislead people into thinking they are making healthy choices. For example, a popular brand of granola cereal has the word "natural" in its name, but contains coconut oil, which contains a high proportion of saturated fat and is loaded with calories. By definition, natural foods are foods that are minimally processed and do not include ingredients such as refined sugars, refined flours, milled grains, hydrogenated oils, sweeteners, food colors, or flavorings.

Opium and horse crap are, by definition, natural too, it doesn't mean that it's good for us or that we would want to ingest it! So by definition, the term "natural" in itself may be technically accurate, but doesn't tell the whole story. You have to read the labels very carefully to get the full picture. Always skip the marketing spin on the front label and go directly to the ingredients list on the back. If you can't pronounce some of the ingredients, then you probably shouldn't be eating them.

These companies try to fool the best of us. Here are some common ways they design to deceive.

1. **Ingredient Splitting**: Using several different types of ingredients, most commonly, sugars combined in a food so they are lower on the ingredients list. As you know, the ingredients list is in order by weight. Food manufactures often use several different forms of sugar—and there are a surprising 40 different types—so they can place them lower on the list, and out of the first three primary ingredients. I have found as many as five types of sugars contained in a single food product, and when their total weight is accounted for, it would have easily been the first ingredient.

2. **Label Padding**: Adding healthy sounding ingredients in small amounts like "acai berry" at the bottom of the ingredients list in order to promote it disproportionately on the front product label.

3. **Unrealistic Serving Sizes:** Some companies list unrealistic amount of servings per container, like one a single serving container of four small cookies and the serving size is 1.3. Who is going to leave that one little cookie behind? It's purely to make the consumer think there are fewer overall calories. Also notorious is sugary beverage containers. Check the label; it may read 2.5 for what looks like a single serving.

It's no wonder we are so confused! To companies who intentionally mislead, I say "BITE ME!" It is up to us to be our own advocates, continually educating ourselves as to what will contribute to our good health, and what will make us sick. Get savvy!

Food Industry Deceptions

Some illusive food manufacturers "spin" their front of package claims to make the product sound better, or healthier for you, than it actually is. They use terms to distract and at times outright deceive. It's up to you to be a savvy food consumer and glean what you can from the information available to you. It's always best to ignore the front of package label and go straight to the nutrition facts, and it's healthiest to avoid processed foods altogether. The claims listed below as "spin" are from actual front of label food products and "the real sin" tells the factual story on from the nutrition panel.

THE SPIN	THE REAL SIN
Tastes like homemade	Unless you made it yourself, it's not homemade
Home-style	Definitely not made at home but in a large factory
Only 4 Carbs!	Yes, low in carbs, but high in saturated fat
Made with REAL eggs	High in cholesterol and saturated fats
100% Natural	May still be high in sugar, calories, fat and sodium
Made with real fruit or fruit juice	Actual percent minimal, loaded with sugars
"0" Trans fat	May be loaded with saturated fat and cholesterol
No sugar added	May be loaded with saturated fat and sugar alcohol
Low Sugar	High potential for fat and sodium
Low Fat	Check for sugar, especially HFCS (High Fructose Corn Syrup)
Reduced Fat	Not low fat, but slightly less than its original full fat version

Made with whole grain	Actual percentage of "whole grain" could be insignificant. Look for "100% whole wheat"
Good source of fiber	May have as little as 2 grams. Goal is 30 g per day
Strengthens your immune system	Meaningless claim, not evaluated by the FDA

Foods That Bite Back

Food products that are labeled in a deceptive manner, with the intention to present the product in a way that seems healthier for the consumer and don't live up to their claims, I consider a Food that Bites Back. The food product below not only makes two misleading claims but also modified the serving size in a grossly unrealistic way.

Non-stick cooking spray

Most of us believe that nonstick cooking spray has zero calories and why wouldn't we? The nutrition facts panel on a poplar non-stick spray makes that claim. One serving is a spray lasting only 1/3 of a second and there are 1057 servings per can. (I challenge you to compress the nozzle for only 1/3 of a second.) What we don't realize is according to FDA law if the "serving size" is less than 5 calories, food manufacturers are permitted to round the calories per serving down to zero. So the serving size is manipulated to a miniscule portion in order to take advantage of this loophole. If you are to moisten your frying pan and spray, say a 4-second spray you may in fact have about 30 calories of canola oil you weren't counting on. The claim on the front of the can states "FOR FAT FREE COOKING". This is clearly not the case. All the calories in this can are derived from fat. The manufacturer further minimizes the claim by stating: Canola oil "ADDS A TRIVIAL AMOUNT OF FAT". Based on their own calculations of a one second spray equaling 7 fat calories, within 5.8 minutes the entire contents of the can will be emptied, totaling 2466 fat calories, and the equivalent weight gain is almost three-quarters of a pound. It is these very deceptive disclosures that hinder out ability to care for ourselves.

While Canola oil in itself is healthy, that is not the heart of the issue. It begs the underlying question "How is it typically used?" I was hosting cook off with many of my clients and teaching them how to prepare foods to minimize the overuse of oils. To displace one of my client's customary methods of deep-frying foods, I asked her to use non-stick cooking spray in its place and to just moisten the bottom of the pan. She used two-thirds of the can to create her dish; the tofu was almost bobbing in oil like an off-shore buoy after a spill. My experience is that most people use it freely without the knowledge of how to use it because they are intentionally mislead and misinformed. The solution, use sparingly. True nutrient profile: 1 gram of fat equals 9 calories per one second spray. A ten second spray is approximately 70 fat calories—hardly a "trivial" amount of fat.

Fast Food InFATuation

"Prayer is the best way to meet the lord. Eating crappy food is faster."

~Toni Julian

Since the McDonalds brothers opened their first burger joint in 1955, Americans have become enamored with fast food. Our need for convenience, in spite of the health risks has become engrained in our lifestyle.

Chef's and food scientists, whether in fast food, high-end, or quick service restaurants, design food to taste delicious, and is typically loaded with all the elements to satisfy our cravings for salt, sugar and fat.

Fast food restaurants strictly fill the need to alleviate hunger but add little to people's nutritional needs. Because each bite of a fast food item is high in salt, sugar and fat, it is extremely calorie dense. Combine this with enormous portion sizes, and the public has been given a skewed sense of what is reasonable which has been source of contention by many over the years. At Rubio's Baja Grill, one of our local quick service mall establishments, you may think you'll be ordering smart by downsizing: a kid's meal includes a cheese quesadilla, chips and a mini-churro and is 900 calories. Add a single refill of a small soft drink for an additional 200 calories. This is more than three times a child needs at one sitting and certainly more than double for an adult!

The poor nutritional values of these meals especially effects teens in terms of weight gain, lack of energy, skin and problems such as breakouts, and even their cognitive abilities. High cholesterol is increasingly present in people in their late teens and early 20's due to the over-consumption of unhealthy convenience foods.

Restaurants that have fewer than 20 locations are now required by law to post their calories and the majority of the larger chains have begrudgingly adhered to this. I have found some people use this as a tool to make healthy selections, while others adamantly state they don't want to know, they want to enjoy their meal and recognize they wouldn't if they were aware their menu item racked up a hefty 1500 calories—almost as many calories as they needed for an entire day! They would rather eat their meal in complete ignorance and bliss!

In spite of nutrition facts postings, some are simply not accurate. Recently, research was conducted to test restaurant claims for accuracy against the actual caloric and fat content of many popular restaurants and in some cases the test results—calculated by a food science lab in Boise, Idaho and gathered from at least eight sources across the country—uncovered incredible obfuscations. For example, Taco Bell posted 4.5 grams of fat for their Grilled Steak Soft Taco, but the test results came back at four times that amount. In another case Macaroni Grill "Pollo Margo Skinny Chicken" was listed as 6 grams of fat by the restaurant however the test results weighed in at a whopping 49 grams of fat. If you continue the logic of that a gram of fat is equivalent to 9 calories, you can see the actual difference in that one macronutrient would be 349 additional calories under-reported for that meal.[4]

I have personally come across a multitude of examples supporting the miscalculations. On a family excursion to Disneyland it occurred to me the likely culprit of such situations; there is a major disconnect between

---

4   Scripps Howard News Service May 2008

the portion sizes stated on the menu, and measured for nutrition information pamphlets, and the chefs who are preparing the food—I call it food creep! Denny's did a marvelous job of scrambling my four egg whites to perfection; the only problem is they served me about eight! And the whole-wheat pancakes that should have been about 3" in diameter were about the same length as my 6-foot 2-inch son's feet. Just because the cooks have quite literally lost sight of portion control doesn't mean you should too.

Many fast food franchises are making an effort to offer more calorically balanced, nutritious meals. McDonalds has re-sized their Happy Meals to more manageable servings—such as a smaller portion of fries—and substituted juice or milk for their sugary soda predecessors and that has helped. Many companies have jumped on the oatmeal bandwagon with hot cereal offerings. A word of caution; simply because oatmeal sounds healthy, like any other food ingredient-- like a baked potato for example--it all depends on how it is prepared. McDonald's oatmeal contains 32 grams of sugar while Jamba has an insulin-spiking 47 grams of sugar. Sadly, the latter nears the equivalent of two Snickers bars at 30 grams each.

FOOD FACTS:
- ✓ Nearly half of our food dollar is spent on food prepared away from home
- ✓ Americans spent $142 billion in 2006 on fast food, as compared to $173 billion on full-service restaurants[5]
- ✓ The US has the largest fast food industry in the world
- ✓ American fast food restaurants are located in over 100 countries[6]

I always find it unsettling when I travel to another country and find one of our fast-food franchises nestled amongst cobblestone streets with Geranium-filled window boxes juxtaposed with the ancient backdrops of the Pantheon and the Roman Forum. Somehow I feel we have violated these cultures with our unhealthy fast foods. Ultimately, these other countries too will pay the price for this infatuation with convenience.

---

5   National Restaurant Association, ND
6   U.S. Bureau of Labor Statistics, Occupational Employment Statistics

CHAPTER 9

JUST SAY "BITE ME!"

"We all need to start making some changes to how our families eat. Now, everyone loves a good Sunday dinner. Me included. And there's nothing wrong with that. The problem is when we eat Sunday dinner Monday through Saturday."

-Michelle Obama

It's time to get real and look at your bad habits straight on. If you watched yourself eat in a mirror would you have gluttony written all over your face?

"BITE ME!" Top 10 Undermining (and Horribly Unattractive) Habits

1. Finishing food from your wife's plate at a restaurant when she's too full to eat her whole meal. That should be your first clue; if she can't finish her own plate, why do you think you should finish hers and yours?
2. Eating the extra serving of mashed potatoes after dinner just so you don't have leftovers. That's just lazy; put them away so you have something to eat when you actually need the extra calories.
3. Cleaning your children's food scraps off their plates. That's what the garbage disposal is for.

4. Even worse, re-eating them after your toddler has spit it out. If you're wondering, "who does that?" go to an amusement park and watch the overweight moms feed their little ones!
5. Licking your fingers after eating ribs to get out all the barbeque sauce from under your fingernails. Think about all the calories you would save if you just used good manners. Towelette anyone?
6. Licking your fingers after eating nachos and popcorn in the movie theater. Your mouth was not made for cleaning. If it was, you'd have been born a cat.
7. Using your tongue to propeller-lick the food off your face. Napkins are square and white and can be found next to the TP at the grocery store.
8. Watching TV while eating mindlessly. If you own a TV tray, ditch it. There is a direct correlation between how many Swanson's TV dinners you've eaten since the 1960's and the width of your butt. There is no technical data on that, it's simply my observation.
9. Inhaling your food. Chew it, slowly, and it may just end up in your stomach rather than your lungs.
10. Skipping breakfast and then hitting the all you can eat buffet, then inhaling your food, then licking your fingers, then eating the food off your kid's plates. You get the point. Eat your breakfast!

Daily Habits

Remember it's the consistent habits we do every day that creates behavior and those habits add up to extra calories! At times we get cravings for something salty, sweet or crunchy and may indulge ourselves by picking up a bag of chips or box of cereal and just mindlessly munch away.

When I was a little girl, I remember my father telling me that it's the small things you do every day that add up to gaining weight. He was an Engineering Manager for FMC, and headed up the project for the Bradley Tank. Every day he went over to the vending machines and bought a small bag of salted peanuts. After about a month of regular visits to Mr. Peanut, he realized he had put on some pounds. Because he did this every day at work, it became part of his routine, that one small snack amounted to extra calories he didn't need on a regular basis. That was my first lesson about weight control. It's okay to have a snack on occasion; it's the daily indulgence that makes the biggest impact.

A couple years ago one of my clients, Sarah, came to me completely frustrated with her weight, as well as the bloating and migraines. I saw her at the gym consistently doing cardiovascular exercises and she wanted to find the cause. I asked her to journal her foods for one week, being sure to measure and even write down the times they were consumed. She had reasonably good eating habits overall, but I knew there was something lurking in those journals that was undermining her ability to lose weight. She had developed a snacking habit at night, after dinner she would crave sugar and fat, and have a cup of trail mix with peanut butter, along with a hot cocoa. There are many reasons contributing to these habits, including eating when we're happy, sad, frustrated or bored. Sarah's situation most likely echoes back to the earlier chapter on uneven blood sugar levels. Eating balanced, small meals throughout the day, our blood sugar levels will even out and we will be less likely to crave and binge on unhealthy foods. When consuming sugary or simple carbohydrate foods, our bodies metabolize it very quickly.

After making the calculations I helped her to realize she was eating over 1000 sugar and fat-laden calories at night, which adds up to a potential weight gain of two pounds every week. We found an alternative for her, a low-fat yogurt and small amount of peanut butter which was not only a much lower calorie substitute but would not create her blood sugar levels to spike. Several weeks later the difference was obvious. She said she was feeling well, no more bloating or struggling with the weight issue.

Some methods to ensure this personal pitfall doesn't sabotage your results are first to keep tempting snack foods out of the kitchen. If you don't buy it, it won't be in your pantry calling to you. Buy a whole grain cereal that you enjoy and rather than snacking out of the box or pouring an endless river into your bowl every morning, pre-portion the servings. I like to check the serving size on the nutrition facts panel, and say its ¾ or one cup per serving; I will measure the entire box into snack baggies and replace them in the original container. This way I have perfectly portioned on the go snack or something to crunch on to satisfy a craving, without the mindless eating.

My personal favorite fix in the evening when I occasionally get a sweet craving is for Good Earth Original Decaffeinated tea. It is naturally sweet and spicy so doesn't need extra enhancements. It warms me up in the wintertime and I drink it iced in the summer. It instantly satisfies any inclinations I have for anything else and hinders my desire to snack.

Excuses, Excuses!

In my lifestyle and nutrition coaching practice, I have heard many well-meaning excuses for why people can't get "started" eating clean. Eating clean, and especially incorporated as incremental lifestyle modifications, happen gradually. It is not some cataclysmic event. If you are waiting for all your stars to align for the "perfect time" that will never happen. You will continue to find excuses for avoiding the best commitment to yourself you can make—your health.

Excuses are simply blocks to prevent you from succeeding. We all make them occasionally. Some blame lack of time, stress, their age, their medical situation, their pasts, or a new job they need to focus on. And while it is easily justifiable in your mind for deferring steps in the right direction, it is ironically the optimal time to take care of yourself. You start simply with choices available to you at the time. You can ask yourself, is this a good food choice, or is there a better one available to me right now? Shall I hit the drive through or pack my lunch the night before? Shall I sit and indulge in these chips in front of the TV, or choose to go on a 20-minute walk? The little choices add up over time to more positive change, improved feelings of well-being and weight loss. As Kathy, one of my clients puts it, "It's contagious!"

Time Management

The all-time worst excuse I have heard is that they don't have time. We're all given the same 24 hours a day, so it comes down to priorities. Whenever someone tells me, "I don't have time," what I hear is, "It's not important to me." We tend to constantly reprioritize given our daily situations and push some activities and goals to the back burner. Usually taking care of ourselves is the first thing we defer.

Lois, my mother who lives in Mexico, asked, "How can you possibly find time to eat five healthy meals a day? It seems your life is so busy, certainly you can't find time to do this!"

My response was "Think of it this way; it is BECAUSE I eat healthy I am able to have a full life and can accomplish all the things I want to do every day!" As I mentioned earlier, we all have the same amount of time in a given day, and it comes down to priorities. We all manage to find the time to do the things that are truly important to us. Feed your body properly, and you will have the nutrients to fuel your day.

Even during my travels to Italy, I found a way to eat small meals five times a day. They weren't optimal, but I never let my blood sugar plummet and was able to stay in homeostasis. My solution was to bring a couple of dozen of my protein-blend muffins—as you will find the recipes for toward the latter part of this book. What made this especially easy is I could bring these food items on the plane along with me, as well as packed them away in my checked luggage.

Taking the opportunity to grocery shop and prepare healthy food also takes time, but I promise you will hit your stride and find it gets easier. What once may have seemed like a chore will become a natural part of your week. You will find that doing a little planning and using the tools in this book, will ultimately leverage your time in the kitchen and you will actually SAVE time in the long run. The payoff will come in the form of feeling great, having more energy and less fatigue because your body will finally be working for you. MAKE time for it in the beginning and it will become habit. It all comes down to priorities.

Stress

Stress in our lives is unavoidable; we all have it at some level. Some of us create stress without realizing it. But if we say we cannot work out or eat well because we're too stressed, we're allowing it to beat us. The stress perpetuates itself as it affects our sleep, our eating patterns, our energy levels, and weakens our immune systems. If we are stressed we may have difficulty falling asleep, or once asleep, wake at 3AM and lay wide-awake, frustrated, until morning. Because we are fatigued, we will tend to self-medicate and eat processed, high carbohydrate foods that will quickly convert to glucose (sugars) in our blood to provide spikes in energy. That's when the insulin comes to the rescue and drives the blood sugar into the cells for storage, creating blood sugar "lows" that can give us headaches and ultimately deplete our energy. We will not feel like working out, in part to the lack of sleep, as well as not having made good food choices to energize our day. You get the picture. Even if you can't do it all perfectly, do as much as you can well to avoid the downward spiral. Seek out stress reduction programs if you feel you need help.

Clients in the midst of making tremendous progress, and are on a path to reach their goals, often encounter stressful situations along the way. My best advice is to go into maintenance mode. When we are overly stressed, and focused on helping a family member get through an illness, or perhaps going through a divorce, you want to make sure you have your primary bases covered.

Some people are very fearful when they encounter a life challenge and the progress they've built may all come crumbling down. Not so with this lifestyle change program. If you have built your strong nutritional foundation, you go back to the basics you've learned: Get enough sleep each night. Eat healthy and frequently throughout the day. Go for walks, being sure to get in at least some exercise. Even if you don't feel like eating, eat small healthy meals anyway (see our no-cooking healthy meal options in Chapter 13 if you're in a pinch). Don't allow yourself to spiral downward. Don't stay in bed with the covers pulled over your head. Get out for a walk, it will help clear your mind and give you energy. Keep the bigger picture in the forefront of your mind.

I had a client who had been telling me she is "ready" for about a year now to start taking care of her. Every time I saw her, she impressed upon me that she is completely frustrated with her weight and is exhausted, trying deprivation diets, working long hours, and multitasking at the expense of her health. She was doing well in our morning fitness program but then decided she needed to take a little time off to get settled in a new job. She was just too stressed. I told her she needed to be *consistent*; this was about fitness and eating well being a part of her lifestyle and she should not give up the tools that are keeping her in a state where she can manage her life in a healthy way. She needed to put herself ahead of all her demands; otherwise she would just go back to her destructive ways of eating and gain the weight she had lost. And that is of course what happened. This stresses the importance of incorporating incremental changes as a part of one's lifestyle, ensuring it is consistent, and not viewing it as a rigid or restrictive diet. Diets are not sustainable. Lifestyle changes you make slowly over the course of your life and keep them in place, and fall back on this structure ESPECIALLY in times of chaos and stress. Eating well and exercising helps you manage your day-to-day challenges and will keep you in a more grounded state.

If you are feeling general stress, then reprioritize your day while keeping your fitness and exercise regimen to the best of your ability. If you decide to let it go, then you are committing to being stressed and not feeling well, which only enables your stress levels to proliferate. If you on the other hand are proactive and hold onto (and value) your good habits you will be in a much better position to deal with the daily stresses that confront you. It is imperative that you help yourself. No one else can make these decisions for you.

Persevere Through Your Past

> "I'm not a victim of my own life, but an orchestrator of my future."
>
> ~ Toni Julian

We can all find reasons to place blame on occurrences in our past, what people may have done to us, or situations we experienced. We need to not live in the past but look forward to our future. Accountability is a character trait that I believe is critical in taking steps to make positive changes in one's life. Without holding ourselves accountable for our own actions, we are not accepting responsibility and are placing blame elsewhere. And if we do that, then we will be ineffective at looking at our situations honestly and making change. Some situations are just out of our control, while others we have brought upon ourselves as a consequence of our action, or perhaps in-action.

I will share some of my life experiences with you, not for sympathy, but so you understand I have been though a multitude of situations that I could have used as excuses, which defer my ability to care for myself. I am sympathetic to the plight of my brothers and sisters, for what everyone has encountered in their lives. Without minimizing difficult pasts, I believe we should strive to take the good out what was there, learn from the bad, and view our lives in a positive light if at all possible—and in some cases look at some situations as blessings. What doesn't kill us makes us stronger, right?

Many years ago, I used to allow my past to define me. By that, I mean I took all my negative experiences and lumped them together in my mind, and viewed myself through this damaged filter, even worse, presented myself to people around me in that way. I believe I was trying to rid myself of the pain of prior childhood experiences, and to reach out and connect, but it never alleviated the hurt or lightened the emotional burden I carried with me.

Today, most of the people I am associated with would be surprised to learn of my background, because I have not let these situations govern who I am today. Most certainly they have helped shaped me, but because they do not DEFINE me, and am able to now be thankful for these experiences and look upon them as contributing to my overall character, I feel stronger and appreciative for them. And when I changed the way I looked at it, I could let go of the pain and the fear. It no longer served me to hold onto it. I'm not a victim of my own life, but an orchestrator of my future.

As children, challenging experiences are especially hard to work as we mature; we are often not equipped to articulate and process what is beyond our years. When I was a young girl our family experienced terrifying events that started when we moved to a farm in Morgan Hill at the end of my 6th grade in Los Gatos.

The old adage about being careful when moving to the country was true, you can encounter some crazy neighbors and unfortunately for us, that is exactly what happened.

The catalyst setting off our un-neighborly dispute had to do with the family living next door. They owned about 10 Pitt Bulls who were bred to fight. They attacked and killed our beloved family dog, Tarzan, an endearing black Lhasa-Apso, escalating into a chain of torrid events. It was illegal to own so many dogs and they barked incessantly through the night for months, causing my mom to come close to a nervous breakdown. When we called the police, they retaliated by spray-painting graffiti on our home. That was simply annoying compared to the string of events to follow. While on a family vacation to Disneyland with my parents and younger siblings, they ran our garden hose through my little brother's bedroom window and literally filled our home with water. My best friend Barb's parents had removed all the furnishings to air dry—we were so grateful for that—and set up fans until our arrival home.

Some months later a military-scale tear gas bomb was thrown into my bedroom window in the middle of the night (when my sister and I were 13 and 14 respectively). In reality, being tear-gassed is not like it is in the movies where you see people cover their faces and cough. The fuming bomb jumps furiously around–most likely designed so the unsuspecting recipients have little ability to catch it and throw it back–emitting fiery flames and a toxic gas in large plumes. Imagine that in a child's 10' x 12' bedroom! When I heard the crash of the canister breaking through the glass of my bedroom window, and looked down from my perch on the upper bunk shared with my younger sister, I tried to scream but could only utter a guttural sound. I was so terrified; I could not find my voice. Suddenly my entire body felt like it was on fire, I felt it first burn my eyes and they began to tear uncontrollably, then my nose began to run, I had trouble breathing and started to choke. I watched the canister bounce around the room, landing on my brand new coat my mom had bought me for the new school year and had carelessly left on the floor before bed.

I recall my panicked parents running in to retrieve us and standing in the cold in the middle of the night in our skimpy night clothes waiting for the ambulance to arrive, shaking and rather snotty. My parents thought all three kids had been accounted for, but my sister decided to run back into the house to retrieve one of our cats. Fortunately, my dad was able to retrieve her unharmed. The firefighters from the El Toro Fire Department burst through the door with hoses, thinking it was a fire. They were yelling "what the hell is that?" not having experienced military-scale tear gas first hand. They came out of the house and were gagging and vomiting near the fire truck.

Imagine sending a family with three kids to the hospital in an ambulance, intentionally. It was insanity. We took showers in the sterile, white-tiled showers at the hospital and I remember how the feeling of water only seemed to make my flesh feel even more seared. We were displaced for about a month, until our home could be cleaned, but it would never be that safe place I once knew. Eventually, all our clothes came back from the cleaners with little white identification tags stapled to every garment we owned and we tried to resume our lives as normally as we could. After settling back into our home, and although the house had been entirely cleaned, we had reminders when we pulled record albums out of their sleeves and were hit with the remnants of the gas, or even years later would come across a small and rude reminder; one of those small white tags on a less-worn shirt or sock.

In fear of further repercussions, my father placed spotlights outside our home to light up our yard so we could see if our not-so-neighborly neighbor intruded into our back yard. We found bullet holes in our door to our kitchen; they had shot the floods out from their yard in the middle of the night. I distinctly recall one Christmas Eve when my dad and I took turns throughout the night until dawn keeping watch. He was very concerned we would be terrorized once again and I felt grown up enough to want to help him take turns at the post. It was the mid 1970's and I was armed with a tape recorder–high tech at the time—and an equally ineffective hand gun. I questioned whether the recorder was useful and whether I would use the gun if I found myself under attack. Fortunately I did not have to decide, they were laying low.

At some point during this two-year long ordeal, the police finally decided to take action to see if they could gather more evidence against our neighbors. Finding the tear-gas bomb clip, along with footprints in the icy lawn to and from their home to my bedroom window was insufficient so they mounted a stake-out. For a couple of nights we had strange men in our home. We kids were told to be very quiet; no one must know that we were home. We learned the operation was less than stealth when the neighbor in question called our home and left a voicemail message that he knew the cops were there.

On April 1, 1976 they burned our home to the ground. I was 16 and was called into the Principals office at school. He was so upset, shaking my shoulders and telling me to stay calm; my house was on fire. He insisted driving me home but I declined, I knew I was fine to drive and he clearly was not. I walked into the house to find nothing but walls remaining. The interior was unrecognizable; the refrigerator was a burned out shell with its charred door gaping ajar. It took me a while to figure out what the orange blob on the floor was and later realized it was the remnants of a melted laundry basket. No one else in my family had arrived home yet. I sat in the back yard amongst the cleared out, blackened debris when my best friend, Barb for whom this book is dedicated, came over after school and found me sitting quietly with the rubble on the back lawn. In shock and disbelief, she asked "Are you okay?" After living through the last year's series of unfortunate events, I realized what was important. My immediate response was "Yeah, I'm fine. Just glad my family wasn't hurt." Even then, I found something to be grateful about.

My father always taught us to reason and get along with people, but that was clearly not in this family's agenda. Eventually we moved back into our rebuilt house, but it was no longer a home without our personal belongings, baby pictures and decorating flare my mom had with antiques. We had lost everything material. My parents divorced and put our home on the market. I remember getting really pissed and yanking the heavy 6' tall "For Sale" post out of the ground and chucking it across the rural road into the creek. I had had enough upheaval with all the hotels and rental homes; I wanted my family together. I didn't want more change.

Once my parents divorced I felt terribly on my own, like there was no one I could rely on. I found a full time job in my junior year of high school and saved money for my future. Because I always took summer school I was able to complete my classes just after my 16th birthday and move on to junior college at 17. I struggled to make ends meet and do well in school. Being so physically depleted, I came down with strep throat, mononucleosis and tonsillitis all at the same time and after a tonsillectomy, because of the scarring, my wounds wouldn't heal and I hemorrhaged. I nearly died that night and was hospitalized for three weeks. After being released, a boyfriend's mother, Marty who has sadly since passed, took me into her home to care for me, making smoothies and sitting me in the beautiful sunshine to heal. I dropped 20 pounds, down to about 95 but eventually made a full recovery. At about that time my mom abandoned her life here in the states and moved to Mexico and has been there ever since.

It was a long haul, seven years to complete my degree while working full time. I had to stay focused, I sacrificed dating or a social life as education was my priority. My teen years taught me some valuable lessons, how to survive and most especially to persevere.
My early life's lessons:

> Take big risks, but make them calculated.
> Reach my goals, make them realistic.
> Invest in myself, do my homework.
> Persevere and be patient, there are no instant results.
> Set myself up for success, not for failure.

It was not by coincidence the words I learned to live by in my early 20's are the same I live by today, and the same words and attitude applies to my outlook and approach to eating. From setting realistic goals to investing in your health through education and coaching, persevering and knowing the only results worth getting and the only results you will keep, are not instantaneous. Set yourself up for success through incremental changes and you won't fail.

Traumatic Events Called Life

Circumstances out of our control are just that, out of our control, but it doesn't mean we have to be flying by the seat of our pants to get through them. Life's ups and downs are inevitable and traumatic situations happen when we least expect them, throwing us off our game.

One of my clients, Colleen, was mid-way through an eight-week lifestyle coaching program when "the bottom fell out" of her life. She was making tremendous progress, eating healthy and committed to "The aabs**Booty**Club™"—our outdoor personalized training program—when her world began to unravel. In a six week period, three family members, her husband, mother, and mother-in-law, all required invasive surgery and she was the primary caregiver charged with nursing them back to health. Because her immune system was compromised she contracted the flu in the midst of all the turmoil. In spite of all these challenges, Colleen kept a positive attitude. She explains:

"Needless to say, I haven't had much time for any focus on myself and I feel like a HUGE failure—both with my workouts and with my eating plan. I was doing great for most of January and early February and then the bottom fell out. You have no idea how frustrating this is for me as I have really been committed to the goal of getting in shape and losing weight. I know it doesn't mean I just can't pick back up again, which is exactly what I will do, but I was making such great strides and the set back has really left me feeling bad. I also know I am somewhat depleted from being a caregiver most of this month and that also takes its toll, but I do feel blessed to have been able to be the support person for my family members. No wonder I got hit with the flu."

Situations like this are so much a part of our lives. We are called upon to be caregivers, supporters, nurturers and nurse-maids, regardless of our own personal level of wellness. At times we may be sick ourselves but still need to provide parenting responsibilities and keep all the many elements of our lives–and those we love—in balance. We are oftentimes the glue that keeps the family together and the safe lap a child needs when life becomes too harsh. But what happens when life happens and the demands of others drown out our inner voice beckoning for balance?

First and foremost we must recognize that in all the chaos, our goal should be adjusted to simply maintaining our fitness and health level.

I suggested this to Colleen as well as making time just to get out in the fresh air for a walk while she is chartered with the task of caregiver. A more recent update from Colleen goes on to explain:

"I'm making a lot of meals, taking my mom to the doctor and physical therapy appointments and general housekeeping for her and my dad. It's actually nice to be spending the time with them. I'm trying to get out for a walk every day this week for about 45 minutes. So far, so good. I think I've maintained and not put any weight on, but since I have not been regular with my Booty Club work outs, I'm afraid I've lost muscle. In the past few weeks, my eating has been off. I crave mostly sugar and simple carbs and have been "mindlessly" eating, grabbing things on the go. I've got clean muffins in the freezer, which I grab, but not all the time. I resort to tortilla chips, pretzels, French bread with butter and cookies, and I'm not paying attention to portion sizes. That's my downfall right now. It just seems like I haven't had the time to pay attention to what I'm eating."

Colleen adjusted her goal and went into maintenance mode. She found opportunities to eat well; she had prepared a healthy stash of protein muffins from recipes in this book so they would be readily available to her and went for walks every day. Surprisingly, she lost about five pounds and made it through her family's crisis in better shape than if she hadn't fallen back on her strong foundation.

Aging and Appreciation

Aging is an inevitable factor which affects our wellness and quality of life. Aging WELL is different than just aging.

Every Sunday afternoon for several hours, my youngest daughter and I volunteer at an assisted living home. We run chair volleyball games and art projects for the elderly. Getting to know this group of people is invaluable; their sincere appreciation comes through every session. Their wisdom is obvious as well as their limitations. The most mobile and fortunate among them have swapped their license to drive a car to trundle behind a high-tech walker. They don't go on brisk walks in the misty morning, they don't bake muffins for their kids, and many have lost their spouse. Most are physically weak with little muscular tone, if any. Some have difficulty remembering my name. I point to my hot pink Nikes and say, "toe," and then to my "knee" in hopes they will recall my name the next time and say "Toni". In spite of these associations the majority have poor memory recall. Some have had strokes, some dementia and others more serious health issues.

It puts my life in a most certain perspective and gives me a strong sense of appreciation for what I am able to do in my life. I always believed that if I used age as an excuse just for the sake of it, I would be yet another obstacle to my success, one in my head. It is never too late to start taking better care of yourself, regardless of your age or level of fitness.

However there is some truth in that we need to modify our eating and fitness regimen as we move through progressive phases of our lives.

As I am learning in my 50's the risk of injury increases exponentially. One major difference is that our tendons and ligaments are less supple, not as elastic as they once were. Our extremities–legs and arms—also have a diminished blood supply so if we are injured it takes longer to heal as it is more difficult for the proteins, nutrients and oxygen in the blood to reach the tendons.

As a result of diminished activity and blood supply we experience a gradual loss of muscle mass. Unless we work on building or maintaining that muscle through exercise—weight bearing activity through the use of weights or your own body weight specifically–we will see a wasting of muscle, loss of strength and are more prone to falls and injury.

In addition, if confined to bed, statistics show people can lose around one percent of muscle strength for each day in bed.

We absolutely must be proactive by incorporating stretching to ensure a full range of motion and flexibility; core training to stabilize our spines, stability and balance training to prevent falls; a healthy diet to keep our minds clear and our bodies nourished; resistance training to keep our muscles toned and bones strong and low impact cardiovascular training (such as walking and hiking) to protect our joints and keep our body burning the fat. The scope of this book does not cover exercise programs and there are many good books and DVD's on the market and online. Just be careful of explosive exercises, those that are fast-paced or include weights not appropriate to your fitness level, and overly strenuous routines; the risk of injury is far greater in advanced-age populations due to the reasons we explained earlier.

About a year ago, my father took a fall. He was stepping up a curb from a parking lot and planted himself shoulder first in a cement bench on the sidewalk, jamming his shoulder and injuring his arm badly. It was my cue to talk with him about balance and stability training. Although he is an avid tennis player, and in great shape, I realized this was an opportunity for him to strengthen his core, to stabilize his body to prevent future falls. I worked with him for a short time and taught him some basic exercises and hooked him up with a personal trainer. After about eight weeks he was able to step onto an elevated step on one leg and balance; a feat he could not have achieved prior. In the following months, he had double knee surgery and his physicians were impressed with his ability to recover so quickly. They attributed it to all the core, balance and stability training he had done for many months before his surgery. So although he was technically "fit" through his tennis games, he had lost some of his core strength along the way. The old adage "use it or lose it" applies and he took it back at close to 80. Appreciate it while you've got it!

CHAPTER 10

MEDICAL ISSUES AND LIVING WITH CHRONIC PAIN

I know some of you reading this have been through worse than I have in either physical or emotional pain; my heart goes out to you and all your hurts. Some of us experience physical pain from injury, aches and pains from obesity and declining physical condition. We remember how our bodies USED to be, how we looked before having kids, or our athletic physique and jean size we wore in high school. I understand the complete frustration and feelings of utter hopelessness and despair. Letting our bodies go to the point where getting to our goal feels so totally far away.

Emotional pain is also devastating and may be hard to recover from entirely. I mentioned the passing of Barb earlier. The emotional toll is heavy; while I have lost my best friend, her mother and father lost their only daughter, her brother lost his sister, her children lost their mother, and her husband lost his wife. I am not sure how I would ever comprehend moving beyond the devastation of such tremendous loss. In the last two years, I've been through as many cancer scares, one for the CIN Cervical Dysplasia, as well as finding a lump in my breast, which after a lumpectomy learned it was benign. I have lived with chronic back pain as a result from a skydiving accident in my 20's, as well as multiple rear-end collisions; one that I am surprised I survived.

As I mentioned earlier, I'm left without a disc between S1 and L5 and pain down both legs from nerve impingement. This threw me for a loop this year and truly tested my fortitude. I am grateful I never turned to pain medications because of the heavy dependence and potential for addiction. Icing, stretching and core exercises have given me some relief, and I continue to work toward a pain free goal. I also have the support of tremendously talented physicians. (Incidentally, the cover photo was taken about a month ago, coming out of my tumultuous year of medical incidents.)

We can choose to make excuses as to why we are the way we are because of it, or use it to make us strong, to make us survivors. I look back and think: I've lived through a lot. Have I suffered all there is to suffer through? Of course not and it's not something I aspire to! I can't pretend to fully understand all individual's suffering, but to the point of this book, to encourage you to do your best, without excuses, to move beyond it and just simply do your best.

Establishing Your Wellness Benchmark

It is always helpful to start with blood work to establish a wellness benchmark and rule out or uncover any medical and hormonal issues so you may have. Simple lab tests can identify hypothyroidism, menopause or Perimenopause, low Grade Infections, high LDL (unhealthy cholesterol), Diabetes and vitamin or mineral deficiencies Some issues may be addressed through nutrition and exercise whereas others may require medications, especially if you have compound problems, such as diabetes plus high cholesterol.

A Walking Time Bomb

Last year I received an email from a woman who was inspired about our story, which ran on the front page of our local newspaper. She desperately wanted to feel better and explained her situation in hopes that I could help.

Soledad explains: "I have come to a point in my life where I am tired of dieting, you know the wrong way: not eating food, starving, drinking shakes and teas then all of a sudden those two pounds that I worked so hard come back with vengeance. After a while I just gave up and just became comfortable with my weight. When I saw your story in the Times I was really inspired. I am 32 years old and would like to lose some weight, just enough to be healthy and so that I can keep up with my very active kids and the restaurant (of course looking good would not be too bad either). I would also like to learn how to keep healthy since I am always on the run and do not have time to cook at home. I feel that my busy schedule is not only affecting me but I have seen the weight gain in my boys since they have been taking advantage of eating at the restaurant."

When we met in person, she said her biggest hindrance was that she ate at a restaurant and was always on the go. Because she spent such a substantial amount of time at work, I recommended she talk with the owner and propose a healthier alternative to add to the menu. She said "I AM the owner" and delighted, I replied, "Then I'm talking to the right person!"

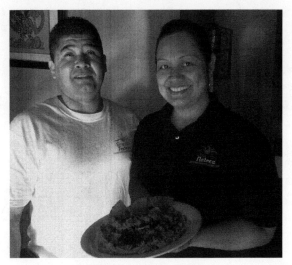

Soledad Quiroz, Age 32
Burrito Azteca, Evergreen Village Square, San Jose, CA

"I was inspired by a front page story about Toni's wellness journey in our local paper and was curious how she had accomplished so

many things after suffering so many health issues. I contacted her and met with her for the first time. Immediately it seemed like we connected on so many levels. Every time I thought of losing weight it seemed that it was such a sacrifice to give up so many good tasting foods and starving. Not so after talking to Toni. She had talked about eating high quality foods, eating clean, and best of all eating frequently. She had suggested seeing a doctor and taking blood work as a place to start, so I could identify potential medical issues right away.

Before I met her, all I did was juggle work and family; I was stressed all the time and ate on the run, mostly fast food. I knew I had to change some of my bad habits. I started as Toni suggested at the doctor's office and was caught off-guard at how many health issues I was faced with. At only 32, I was anemic, had a chronic sinus infection, fibroids in my uterus, high cholesterol, border-line diabetes, low blood pressure, and of course over-weight. The doctor was really concerned about all these issues but he was most concerned about my weight and the high cholesterol since that could be life threatening—especially given the amount of stress that I was dealing with on a day to day basis. I was what he called "a walking time bomb".

My grandmother just passed away February 14, 2010 and with her, a big part of our selves was lost as we were so close to her. This really changed my way of thinking. Did I want to ignore my health issues and leave my loved ones in pain because of my poor bad habits? Worst of all did I want my kids to learn these nasty habits?

I finally made the decision and started making baby steps towards better lifestyle changes. I try to make simple modifications in my eating habits and try not to eat out as much. Toni came to our restaurant and created a dish that became the foundation of my understanding to healthy clean food. I slowly began to feel an improvement in my health.

Mostly importantly, I lost 10 pounds and was able to get pregnant after years of trying and the doctor had told me it was going to be close to impossible.

Today I see many small changes in my family and my kids. We see the doctor more regularly for check-ups, I read food labels, cook with less oil, focus on eating clean, and am now aware of bad habits. The best part of this is my family now knows the direct consequences of eating poorly, which is bad health!"

Soledad, and her husband Adrian, have made a brave commitment by stepping out of their comfort zones and learning how to prepare and bring healthy options to the community. Soledad took the initiative to get blood work and understand her wellness benchmark, is now four months pregnant and has become a healthier role model for her family as well!

Critical Health Numbers

Critical health numbers are as imperative to know as their name implies. Physicians recommend you have tests performed periodically so you have the information you need to ascertain your level of wellness. What may be on the outside is not always a good indicator of what's going on a physiological level.

Create a baseline now, so you can test your levels in a few months to track the changes after you've established a clean-eating regimen. You will be able to see the difference it makes not only on the outside, but the inside!

Simple tests can be performed to check your blood pressure, and getting weighed weekly on your bathroom scale helps keep tabs on your body weight. Lab tests can disclose a multitude of issues you may not even be aware of such as vitamin deficiencies, low grade infections, high cholesterol or low fasting blood sugar levels.

Studies have shown that 80% of the US population is deficient in vitamin D and the majority of us rarely get all the nutrients we need. Show your doctor this book, the healthy changes you are making, and talk about potential supplementation if necessary. Most of us need to have a multivitamin, vitamin D, calcium and the right balance of Omega 3 to Omega 6 fatty acids; fish oil or flaxseed meal are good sources.

Here is a partial list of tests as a starting place (check with your doctor to see which ones are relevant for you and for others not on this list). For more information on critical health numbers go to the American Heart Association at www.heart.org.

Test	Method	What is being measured
Scale/Monitor Tests		
Weight	Scale	Total Body Weight
Body Composition	Hydrostatic Immersion	Actual Body Fat and Lean Mass
Blood Pressure	Blood Pressure Monitor	
Lab Tests		
Blood Sugar	Glucose Test	
Blood Cholesterol	Blood Lipid Profile	HDL-High Density Lipoprotein
		LDL-Low Density Lipoprotein
Vitamin D	Blood Test	
Thyroid Panel	Blood Test	T3 and T4 Free, TSH (Thyroid Stimulating Hormone)
Hormones	Blood Test	FSH (Follicle Stimulating Hormone)
		Progesterone, Testosterone, Estradiol
Blood Cell Count	Blood Test	White Cell Count, Red Cell Count
Anemia	Blood Test	Iron deficiency
Procedures		
Colonoscopy	Procedure	Colon
Mammogram	X-Ray Procedure	Identifying irregular breast mass
Breast Exam	Self-Check at Home	Locating lumps or cysts
Prostate	Physician Exam	Check for enlargement

Important Tips:

- Always go to the same lab as results can vary slightly among the different diagnostic companies.
- Do your part to ensure accurate results by following the preparation instructions, such as fasting for Glucose testing for Diabetes or cleaning out your plumbing prior to a colonoscopy! Drink plenty of water if you are having blood drawn.
- At the time of your appointment with the lab request copies of your results to be distributed, not only to the physician who ordered the tests, but to your OB/GYN, primary care physician and other specialists.
- Keep yourself in the loop. Always request a copy for your personal file.
- Ask your physician to review and more importantly, interpret the results in person with you and watch for trends.
- If there are results that fall in abnormally high or low ranges, ask your physician how often you should have follow up lab work to track your progress or keep tabs on a situation that needs watching.
- BE YOUR OWN ADVOCATE. ASK QUESTIONS. OWN THE PROCESS. IF YOU NEED HELP, ASK A FAMILY MEMBER OR FRIEND.

The Complexities of Medication

I would be remiss if I did not mention the use of medications in this chapter. I was in a fog on just a handful of different medications. Some people I know are on 25 or 30 different prescription medications and walk around in a stupor. Some medications are necessary and required. Our life may depend on them. Other times they help us with some annoying symptoms, some may have had their place a decade ago, but we are still on them out of habit, while others are not necessary at all. Some people do fine on certain medications while others have an idiosyncratic reaction; that is an unusual response to a medication that others may not experience.

Physicians are caught in a quandary. Patients get frustrated being told they need to exercise, or eat right, or cut out the Angus cheeseburgers, reduce salt, eat their fruits and vegetables, and drop some weight.

Perhaps in their heart they know they should but they want a simple solution so physicians oblige them with a prescription that serves to alleviate the symptom, not remedy the actual cause. I recall a survey that showed the overwhelming majority of patients who went to the doctor were more satisfied when a prescription was given to them then when simply given lifestyle change advice. We as patients help drive this propensity to over prescribe. As part of a $122 billion dollar industry, pharmaceutical companies have agendas as well and spend $2.5 billion per year on advertising and pull-through marketing campaigns, to make their drugs household names and encourage you to ask your doctor about their particular medication.

Be aware of biases when it comes to prescriptions and OTC medications. If there is a lifestyle solution or dietary change to resolve the problem, talk to your doctor about it. If your physician suggests medication, think it through and do your research because everything you put in your mouth; food, prescriptions, supplements and over the counter medications, makes a significant impact on your health–for better or worse. And as you read in my own life experience, the side effects were devastating and completely avoidable.

If you are not proactive with your health, and if you are not sleeping and eating right, if you are overweight and do not take care of yourself, you are much more likely to develop diabetes, high blood pressure, some forms of cancer, stroke or cardiac issues, and the medication is sure to follow. The real answer is be proactive, take care of yourself now so you can stave off disease, or at least be in a better, stronger position to fight it.

Some tips when evaluating if a medication is right for you:
Ask yourself and your doctor:

- ✓ Do the benefits outweigh the risks?
- ✓ What are the potential side effects?
- ✓ Is this medication addictive (especially for pain medications)?
- ✓ Am I taking other medications that have the potential to intensify side-effects?
- ✓ Is there a more natural way to heal myself?
- ✓ If I improve my lifestyle will I need this medication long-term?

When taking medications:

- ✓ Keep a journal of the name, dosage, and how often you take it.
- ✓ Make sure only one physician is in charge of managing your prescriptions.
- ✓ Always share your prescription information with all other physicians you are seeing.
- ✓ When a new medication is prescribed, always ask your doctor if it will have any negative drug interactions with your other medications, both prescription and OTC (over the counter).
- ✓ Let a family member or your emergency contact know what you are taking and where the medications are located in your home.
- ✓ Bring your journal with you to all medical appointments so you can refer to it with your physician. (Be sure to log any tests, lab work and comments or instructions by your doctor.)

CHAPTER 11

LEARN TO EAT CLEAN

What is clean eating? I am asked that on a daily basis. As opposed to what, "dirty eating?" It's not an intelligently intuitive phrase, but I suspect it's derived by the way it makes your body feel . . . . clean, strong and in homeostatic balance! It's a term that's been around for years in the fitness industry, but is not too well known yet by the general public. I frequently give seminars on the topic and typically not one person in the room is familiar with the term. It's an education process, and anyone who has heard of clean eating is ahead of the curve. The benefits are substantial; when you eat clean, your body will feel light, energetic and healthy. With the added nutrients your hair will be shinier and will grow faster, your complexion will clear, and even your nails will become stronger; your mind clearer as the fog of inflammatory foods will be lifted.

Eating clean is eating whole foods, as close to their original form as possible and minimizing foods that come with a Nutrition Facts panel unless it is made with whole, natural foods and minimally processed. Whole foods can include fresh fruits, vegetables, whole grains, and lean meat, nuts, seeds, beans and dairy.

10 Quick Tips for Healthy, Clean Eating

1. Eat breakfast to boost your metabolism. If you skip this important meal, you will be setting yourself up for failure for the rest of the day.
2. Eating small meals every two to three hours is imperative to maintaining a high metabolism. Eating five to six small meals a day evens out your blood sugar and provides the necessary fuel throughout your day.
3. Make your meals at home rather than eating out so you know what you're eating. Research has shown we under-estimate the caloric values of our meals eaten out by 50%!
4. Stick with natural foods, as close as possible to its original form, like a whole apple, rather than sweetened processed applesauce.
5. Stay away from processed foods; they typically have added sugars, sodium, fats and chemicals and are stripped of many nutrients.
6. Combine protein and complex carbohydrate at each meal. Think 20/60/20 ratio of protein/complex carbohydrates/ healthy fats.
7. Plan snacks and meals ahead of time and bring them with you so you don't resort to unhealthy alternatives.
8. Use a slight amount of olive and canola oils when cooking, just enough to moisten the bottom of the pan with a napkin or paper towel. Even better, use nonstick cooking spray in either of those two varieties.
9. Always broil, boil, poach, grill or toast (without butter). Completely avoid fried foods.
10. Finally, give your taste buds a chance to adjust to wholesome foods again. If you are accustomed to cream sauces, butter-saturated movie theater popcorn or find it necessary to dip your tortilla chips into processed cheese spread, allow your buds a little extra time!

Clean Meal Solutions

The CLEAN meal solutions in this book have been specifically designed to be simple to prepare, using fresh, nutritious foods and convenient and accessible pantry foods. The concept is to make healthy foods your new convenience foods. The vast majority of these recipes have the perfect blend of protein, carbohydrates, and healthy fats so they are balanced to keep you satiated and provide the nutrients you need all day. Make each bite work in your best interest!

More than just a recipe book, this is a lifestyle book. It's filled with tools you can apply to your busy life in a way that is realistic, simple AND inspirational. Leveraging your time in the kitchen—through using these recipes for multiple meals, having nutritious foods available and on the go, and freezable options for quick meal fixes—will allow you to provide nourishing meals that are as healthy as they are good-tasting.

I have developed them all from scratch, use them to fuel our family, and know they make efficient use of my time because I use them personally, on a daily basis. The beauty of these foods is that you can eat any of them at any time of the day.

Benefits of Clean Eating—From the Inside, Out!

After my clients have changed their eating habits to what they call "BITE ME!" habits, some of their health issues are reversed or at least minimized, from annoying menopausal symptoms to Diabetes to high cholesterol levels. They have taken control of their bodies and minimized their risk factors for disease. Energy levels are increased, weight and blood pressure is reduced, and their lab work gives them tangible results that make them so proud they want to post it on Facebook, or at least on their refrigerator door.

Norma, one of my lifestyle coaching clients, is a bright, professional, 51 year old woman who found me through some mutual friends. We had gone to high school together and hadn't seen each other in over 30 years. I remembered her as the bouncy and energetic cheerleader with amazing muscular legs! In spite of her popularity she was also kind to everyone around her. She came to me a couple of months ago and said she felt that she strongly wanted to "make a big change in my body and my lifestyle." During my first meeting with her we were both teary-eyed; I could feel her frustration within herself and listened as she explained her life situation. Standing at just a little over 5' tall, she had found herself about 50 pounds overweight, and genetically carried it primarily around her middle; momentum fat is associated with several health risks so I was genuinely concerned. She was on medication for Diabetes and felt lethargic. Given her poor diet and lack of consistent exercise due to a recent move and other stressors, she came to realize she had little time remaining in her day for herself and felt miserable.

I was immediately impressed with Norma when she came to me with a realistic approach. Instead of asking me to put her on a diet, or that she wanted to lose a large amount of pounds by a certain timeframe, she intuitively wanted to make lifestyle changes, was concerned about her health issues, and asked me how long it might take for her to accomplish her goal. Between her diligent efforts of better eating choices, and adding walking and cardio to her day, she went from 42% body fat down to 34% in the first five weeks; a change of 9% in her body composition.

Norma shifted the priority to herself; transitioning to cleaner-eating habits, making foods for herself and avoiding the fast foods. Under the care of her physician, she was able to reduce her Diabetes medication by half and is on the way to weaning herself off completely. She even declared her office area a "NO CANDY ZONE" to avoid temptation. She continues to strive to hit her goal, which I am sure she will reach within the next few months. I'm so very proud of her diligence!

How to Select the Correct Foods

Whether you are making a meal from a recipe or just grabbing left over foods a la carte, you will want to make sure you have the correct balance of lean proteins, complex carbohydrates and healthy fats. As mentioned before, this helps stabilize your blood sugar levels, increases satiety and provides better nutrition through variety. Over the years I have developed a list of all the healthy, nutritious foods found in my recipes to make shopping easier and more importantly, to give ideas when I feel I am fresh out of them! Studies have shown that most Americans buy the same five fruits and vegetables every time we go to the store. How boring is that?

In general:

- ✓ Chose complex carbohydrates, including whole grains, like 100% whole wheat breads, pitas, pastas and tortillas, quinoa, brown rice, oats and barley.
- ✓ Eat lean proteins, such as fish, egg whites (limit the yolks, they are high in cholesterol), chicken breasts, pork tenderloin, lean ground turkey and nonfat dairy or a combination of rice and beans (rice and beans contain all the essential amino acids and therefore create a complete protein).
- ✓ Include small amounts of raw nuts and seeds, such as almonds, walnuts, sunflower and pumpkin seeds.
- ✓ Focus on fresh organic fruits and vegetables, as many varieties and colors as you find, making your plate look like a work of art.
- ✓ Include dairy, such as nonfat plain yogurts, non-fat or low-fat cottage cheese, and nonfat milk, or whey protein for convenience.

Building Your Meal

Let's get down to the details. To balance your meals you will find the list below of healthy options. Note they are broken down into categories one through six.

Category 1	PROTEINS
Categories 2, 3 and 4	CARBOHYDRATES
Category 5	HEALTHY FATS
Category 6	CONDIMENTS AND HERBS

ACTION	EXAMPLE
Select a lean protein from category 1:	3 oz Chicken Breast
Select a carbohydrate from 2, 3 or 4:	1 cup Sweet Potato
Select a healthy fat from category 5:	10 Raw Almonds
Select a condiment from category 6:	Cinnamon and Cumin rub for Chicken

Now that you have achieved balance, note the portion size for each food. The list breaks down healthy serving sizes for each food. You may need to modify the servings upward slightly if you need more calories overall.

Also note the ballpark calories for each serving at the top of each category. You can keep mental track when planning to hit your target of 250 to 350 calories per meal, depending upon your goals. The calories per item are not exact! For example, a medium apple is 80 calories although I am estimating it at 100. I am rounding so you can make simple equations without having to search for your calculus calculator every time you eat.

When it comes to menu planning, look at the recipes as tools. They are already balanced for you nutritionally and calorically. Or, build your own meal using the template below.

Many nutrition or diet books will lay out a 30 day eating plan for you however you will not find that approach in this book. I want you to learn for yourself what to eat and when. I want you to be accountable for the decisions you make. I want to make it easier for you to prepare and select your foods. Decades ago, when I tried "dieting" I followed specific plans that detailed every ingredient I needed to eat breakfast, lunch and dinner for weeks on end. I wound up with a refrigerator full of food that I could not possibly eat during the week, and worked way too hard to have every ingredient the meal called for on a particular day. If I didn't have the "pita" or the "1/2 orange" I would feel like I had failed. It was exhausting. So be creative choosing your foods, find balance, eat the right portions and it will all become second nature to you soon.

MENU PLANNING: TARGET CALORIES PER MEAL: 250-350

IDEAS FOR BALANCED MEALS:

Items	Categories	Calories
Ground Turkey+Spinach+Pasta	1+3+4	6 meals x 250 calories = 1500 cal
Whey Protein+Blueberries+Flaxseed	1+2+5	6 meals x 300 calories = 1800 cal
Cottage Cheese+Pineapple+Almonds	1+2+5	6 meals x 350 calories = 2100 cal
NF Milk + Oatmeal +Banana	1+4+2	5 meals x 350 calories = 1750 cal

CATEGORY 1			CATEGORY 2		
Lean Proteins			**Fruits**		
About 150 Calories Per Serving			About 100 Calories Per Serving		
3	oz	Chicken Breast	1	cup	Black Cherries
1	serving	Whey Protein Powder	1	item	Plum
1	serving	Soy Protein Powder	1	item	Grapefruit
3	oz	Turkey Breast	1	item	Peach
3	oz	Bison	1	Serv*	Dried Apricots
3	oz	Lean Ground Turkey	1	item	Apple
3	oz	Pork Tenderloin	1	item	Pear
		Fish	1	cup	Grapes
5	oz	Cod	1	item	Orange
5	oz	Halibut	1	item	Banana
3	oz	Salmon	1	T	Dried Cranberries
3	oz	Scallops	1	item	Pomegranate
3	oz	Shrimp	1	cup	Blueberries
5	oz	Tuna	1	item	Tomato
5	oz	White Fish	1	cup	Cantaloupe
			1	item	Nectarine
		Dairy	1	item	Kiwi
			1	cup	Strawberries
About 100 Calories Per Serving			1	cup	Blackberries
1	cup	Nonfat Plain Yogurt	1	cup	Pineapple
1	cup	Soy Milk	1	cup	Unsweetened Applesauce
1	cup	Nonfat Milk	1	cup	Raspberries
1	cup	Nonfat Cottage Cheese	1	Serv*	Raisins
1	cup	Egg Whites	*For dried fruit, always check package for portion size and watch for added sugars		

CATEGORY 3			CATEGORY 4		
Vegetables			**Grains**		
About 50 Calories Per Serving			About 200 Calories Per Serving		
1	cup	Artichokes	1	cup	Pearled Barley
1	cup	Asparagus	1	cup	Bulgur
1	cup	Broccoli	2	slice	Whole Wheat Bread
1	cup	Beets	1	cup	Brown Rice
1	cup	Cauliflower	2	oz	Whole Wheat Pasta
1	cup	Celery	1	item	Whole Grain Tortilla
1	cup	Cucumbers	1	cup	Quinoa
1	cup	Eggplant	1	cup	Oatmeal
1	cup	Green Beans	2	T	Wheat Germ
1	cup	Romaine Lettuce	1	item	Whole Wheat Pita
1	cup	Peppers, all varieties	1	item	Whole Wheat Bagel
1	cup	Snow Peas	1	Serv	Whole Grain Cereal
1	cup	Spinach			*1 serving of uncooked grains is approx ½ cup, cooked is 1 cup
1	cup	Young Summer Squash	**Beans**		
1	cup	Zucchini			*1 serving of beans uncooked is ¼ cup dry
1	cup	Dried Peas	1/4	cup	Black Beans
1	cup	Baby Lima Beans	1/4	cup	Pinto Beans
1	cup	Carrots, cooked	1/4	cup	Kidney Beans
1	cup	Green Peas	1/4	cup	Yellow Split Peas
1	cup	Bok Choy	1/4	cup	Lentils
1	item	Corn on the Cob	1/4	cup	Green Split Peas
1	cup	Canned Pumpkin	1/4	cup	Black Eye Peas
1	Serv	Onions	1/4	cup	Small Red Beans
1	Serv	Garlic	1/4	cup	Great Northern Beans
1	T	Hummus	1/4	cup	Lima Beans
1	cup	Sweet Potato or Yam	1/4	cup	Small White Beans

CATEGORY 5			CATEGORY 6	
Fats (About 100 Calories per Tablespoon)			**Condiments and Herbs**	
1	T	Olive Oil	(FREE!)	
1	T	Flaxseed Meal		
1	T	Avocado	Mustard	
1	3 sec	Nonstick Cooking Spray	Chicken Broth (low sodium)	

		Nuts/Seeds			Nutmeg
1	Serv	Peanuts	*1 Serving of nuts or seeds is approx one tablespoon		Chinese 5 Spice
1	Serv	Pumpkin Seeds			Allspice
5	Item	Raw Almonds			Nutmeg
1	Serv	Raw Walnuts			Cinnamon
1	Serv	Almond Butter			Cumin
1	Serv	Peanut Butter			Oregano, Parsley, Cilantro, etc.

What clean eating is NOT: Overly processed foods where the nutrients have been stripped, such as foods made with white flour such as pizza dough, doughnuts, cookies, and pastries; saturated artery clogging fats that lurk in bacon and sausages, heavy cream and butter sauces, and fast foods devoid of nutrients and fiber, and high in saturated fat and calories; foods that are sugar laden, with added corn syrups. Processed meats such as bacon, deli-meat, hot dogs and sausages containing nitrites (chemicals to make the meats appear red) and Heaven forbid the combination of sugary, fried, processed foods. Clean eating is also minimizing alcohol consumption. All these defy clean eating habits, will throw your body in homeostatic imbalance, and undermine your health, not to mention your physique.

Supplementation

Recently a new client, who I'll call Carrie, shared her eating program with me. She had it neatly typed out in an Excel format; meticulously laying out the details including quantities, time she ate and type of food. Her journal was loaded with tea powders, protein shakes, fiber additives, aloe extracts, artificial sugars, glutamine powders, BCAA's, vegetable powders, drink mixes, and "fat burning spices." My first questions were, "Where's the REAL food?" and, "How do you know if these are even working?"

Her diet was constructed by a nutritionist, so what little real food she was eating was at least healthy. She was on a carbohydrate cycling plan so that her blood sugars were very low several days a week, followed by a high-carb day. She ate exactly the same foods every day, without variation and excluded the fruit she needed from a nutritional standpoint. I asked her how this was sustainable for her as the calories were restricted so severely, and she commented she had been on much more rigid diets in the past and that she could sustain it. She was extremely "compliant" when it came to following this specific program, showed much more determination and willpower than most anyone I had met, however the nutritional sustainability was unhealthy. Worse yet, she felt terrible, had low energy and was not getting the results she needed—a change in her body composition, working toward reducing fat and increasing muscle mass.

Nutrition is the single most important part of everyone's vitality and a healthy program should be built around a strong nutritional foundation. In other words, design your life around healthy REAL food and not supplements. I consider supplements to be any form of processed protein shakes, bars, pills and powders used to round out an already balanced diet. Supplements could also mean vitamin supplements for specific deficiencies, however the purpose of our conversation here is targeted toward the overwhelming oversupply of a non-FDA regulated, supplemental industry that essentially makes any claim they desire. Supplements are typically very expensive and recommenders have financial gains to be made without evidence of a benefit. They often tout "research" that proves their product fights cancer and with the stamp of approval from a doctor, people swallow the whole story, so to speak. Always find out who has conducted the research; if the company manufactured the supplement and conducts its own research, that's not research, its marketing. That said there are many good quality supplements, and many that are a complete waste of money. The important thing is determining which are best.

Our lifestyle sometimes makes it difficult for most of us to eat five or six REAL meals a day, consisting on lean proteins, complex carbohydrates and healthy fats—and avoiding processed or fast foods—so supplementation has its place. Keep in mind a protein powder or bar is not at the highest level of food quality so it should be used no more than one time a day to take the place of one of your five or six meals from a convenience standpoint. We should not subsist on supplements first, nor should they be given an equal share in your diet.

They are never as good as the "real thing" and are not metabolized as well as natural, organic foods.

The only situation where supplementation makes sense: If you have no time for a meal and your healthiest option is a protein bar or shake versus your potential options, such as a burger and fries.

Vitamins and essential lipid supplements, on the other hand, when needed to compensate for deficiencies, are completely another matter. A liquid multi-vitamin can cover your bases and is easily absorbed. Most Americans are deficient in Vitamin D, and unless you are eating fish four or five days a week, such as Salmon or Orange Roughy, or consuming flax seed, you will need an Omega-3 fatty acid. Women require calcium supplementation, and the requirements increase post-menopause.

Your blood work will also show any other deficiencies, such as potassium or iron that you may also need to supplement. The goal is to build a strong foundation by getting the majority of your nutrition from REAL food and supplement as needed.

CHAPTER 12

LET'S GET ORGANIZED!

My guess is you would very much like to succeed at incorporating healthier eating habits into your lifestyle so that makes two of us. And unless you'd like to see this book end up as a margarita coaster on your coffee table, it's time to get organized. You've heard the saying, "If you fail to plan then you plan to fail," so let's get to it.

Using a combination of meal solutions provided in this book, along with easy, no-cook options, the perfect balance of protein, carbohydrates and healthy fats is achievable every day by incorporating fruits, vegetables, lean proteins and grains for each meal. Most any meal solution in this book will net a healthy balance by the end of the day. Check out the following example based on 1500 total calories and allows room for the addition of healthy nuts and seeds.

Observe the following:

- ✓ There are five meals spread throughout the day.
- ✓ Each meal has the proper balance of nutrients
- ✓ The calories are divided generally equally between all the meals.
- ✓ Meals and snacks should be treated the same, regardless of whether you call them an actual meal or snack.

Sample Daily Menu—Based on 1500 calories per day

(You will adjust yours higher depending upon your individual needs)

	Protein	Carbs	Fat	Calories
Breakfast				
Apple-Cinnamon Multi-Grain Oatmeal	8	30	4	178
AM Snack				
BITE ME! Banana Nut Muffins	17.5	58	4.5	330
Lunch				
Grilled Chicken Breast with Mango Salsa & Pita Chips Fresh Spinach	39	32	6.4	357
PM Snack				
½ Cup Blueberries				
One Half Cup Cottage Cheese, 1%				
One Serving Kashi GoLEAN Cereal	22.3	52	2.7	283
Dinner				
Serving Parmesan Turkey Meatballs with Spaghetti				
Van Gough Veggie Salad	27.6	56	4.4	376

Total Percent of Calories from:

Protein 29% 128g

Carbs 57% 256g

Total Fat 14% 27g

Saturated Fat 5g

Weekly To-Do List

Here's a quick tip list for starting each week. Sundays seem to work best for most of my clients but choose a day when you have a few hours prior to the start of your week.

✓ Select a few meals to prepare from this book
✓ Make your grocery list and shop
✓ Make your meals on a day off and place them in individual containers for quick heating over the next few days. Freeze a few for later in the week.
✓ Schedule your walks, hikes, bike rides or gym workouts for the week.

Five-Fork Rating

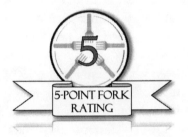

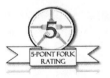 When you are grocery shopping, be sure to buy the highest quality ingredients available. Here's a FIVE POINT FORK system for you to use to determine which foods are best. Give your food a point for each criterion met. The more forks, the better the quality and better results you will achieve by fueling your body with essential nutrients.

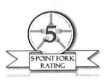 Completely Unprocessed: As close to their original source, essentially foods that are unaltered and contain only one ingredient, such as a fruits, vegetables, legumes, lean meats, nuts and seeds.

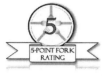

Low Sodium: Foods without added sodium chloride. Avoid canned vegetables, soups and sauces. Check labels on frozen vegetables for added salt.

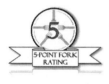

Low Fat, Zero Trans Fat, Zero Saturated Fat: Foods that contain no unhealthy fats, especially those found in red meats and any fat that is firm at room temperature. Also check percentage of calories from fat: 1 gram or less of fat per 50 calories is a good rule of thumb when selecting processed foods to keep you in the roughly 20-30% range of calories derived from fats. Stick to unsaturated fats and shoot for zero trans-fats or saturated fats. Although nuts, seeds, avocados and olive oils contain fats, the LDL (Low Density Lipoproteins) fats offer valuable health benefits. Eat them in moderation as they are calorie dense.

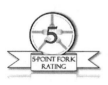

Low Sugar: Foods (excluding fresh fruits) that contain less than 4 grams of sugar—in any form such as brown sugar, white granulated, corn syrup, fructose, etcetera per serving.

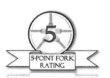

Organic and Locally Grown: Natural foods free of pesticides and chemicals and grown in your community are the freshest and picked closer to their peak ripeness. Hit those Farmers Markets!

"BITE ME!" Grocery List

Your grocery shopping just got easier. All ingredients from the recipes are included in this immediately downloadable, Excel-format grocery list. Customize by adding your own foods you and your family use to make it all-inclusive. Never run out of the necessary staples for your favorite recipes or quick healthy foods for snacks by putting it on your refrigerator door. As soon as you're running low or used the last of an item, simply check it on your list. It's consolidated and an easy reminder. Send an email to info@aabs.us.com for your free downloadable grocery list.

Necessary Kitchen Tools

- ✓ Food Chopper
- ✓ Food Processor/Grater
- ✓ Blender
- ✓ Mixer
- ✓ Waffle Iron
- ✓ Electric Grill
- ✓ Electric Tea Pot
- ✓ Crock Pot
- ✓ Rice Cooker
- ✓ Measuring Spoons
- ✓ Easy View Measuring Cups

The Perfect Pantry

An ideal pantry is one that has all your staples readily available for making clean meals. So it's time to purge the pantry of all your hidden stashes and nasty nibbles that will take you off track. Trash the chips and instant cake mixes, the white flour and two year old sugar cones. Cleaning your pantry will make you feel good all under.

Measure your cabinets and purchase pop-top, stacking canisters of assorted heights and sizes, the type with the button on top that creates a vacuum and seals your foods.

Cut the nutrition facts panel from the original package and place it inside the front of the canister, facing out, then fill it with the appropriate contents. The food will hold the label in place and you'll always have access to this valuable information.

Identify each canister with removable, laminated label. Here are some key ingredients to a BITE ME! regimen.

- ✓ Flaxseed Meal
- ✓ Whole Wheat Flour
- ✓ Raw Almonds
- ✓ Dried Walnuts
- ✓ Raw Sunflower Seeds
- ✓ Brown Rice
- ✓ Oat Bran
- ✓ Oat Flour
- ✓ Steel Cut Oats
- ✓ Mixed Dried Beans
- ✓ Polenta
- ✓ Quinoa
- ✓ Barley
- ✓ Dried Fruits (without added sugars)

CHAPTER 13

THE ONLY REASON I HAVE A KITCHEN IS IT CAME WITH THE HOUSE WHEN I BOUGHT IT

No-Cooking-Required-Meal Solutions

If the only reason you have a kitchen is because it came with the house when you bought it, this section is for you. Here are some ideas to pack nutrition and convenience into your day. All meals are around or under 300 calories with minor preparation or designed to be made in advance and used for on-the-go situations.

- ✓ ½ cup low fat or non fat cottage cheese with 1/2 cup of Kashi GoLean cereal and ½ cup blueberries
- ✓ Edamame (soy beans)
- ✓ Sliced green apples, 1 tablespoon almond or other natural nut butter and brown rice cake
- ✓ ½ 100% whole wheat pita with 2 tablespoons Healthy Hummus and handful of red bell pepper slices
- ✓ Low fat plain yogurt mixed with 1 tablespoon PB2 and one banana
- ✓ ¼ cup BITE ME! Trail Blazin' Stash with handful of baby carrots

✓ The Quickie Smoothie: ½ cup berries, 1 cup nonfat milk or soy or rice dream, 1 scoop protein powder, 6 raw almonds and a few ice cubes. You can substitute any frozen or fresh fruit.

✓ Mini Pizzas: 100% whole wheat English muffin, organic tomato sauce, 1 tablespoon shredded light mozzarella cheese, fresh mushrooms and spinach leaves. Broil in oven until toasty.

✓ Three eggs scrambled (only 1 yolk) in 100% whole-wheat tortilla with any leftover steamed veggies and topped with salsa. Can be made in microwave or pan.

Restaurant Ordering Tips

Over 50% of our food dollar is spent on restaurants and the average American eats out at least four times each week. Although restaurants are required to post their calorie breakdowns, recent research has shown that some caloric facts are misrepresented and understated by as much as five times! I would encourage you to eat primarily at home or pack your foods to take on the road with you. Knowing what you are eating is key to a healthy lifestyle! If you need to eat out, be certain to order your foods selectively. Here are some tips when ordering:

1. **Don't be shy about asking for what you want, you just might get it.** Our family was on a trip recently and the consensus was to go to the Jack in the Box drive through. I ordered the healthiest item on the menu, the Chicken Teriyaki Bowl. I specified "no sauce" and "double steamed vegetables". I was pleasantly surprised when my bowl was packed with lean chicken chunks, white rice (not brown, but not bad) and an enormous helping of steamed assorted vegetables. SCORE!

2. **Build Your Meal to Build Your Metabolism:** Design your meal to include a healthy balance of lean protein, complex carbohydrates and healthy fats. Scan the menu for simple foods where the preparation can be modified or you can ask for substitutions.

> Focus on your protein first, asking for lean cuts of chicken (skinless), fish or pork tenderloin, preferably grilled or poached. Be sure to request "no butter or oils" used in the grilling process.

(Some restaurants will add an enormous pat of butter to their steaks and chicken.

Next, choose a complex carbohydrate if available, such as brown rice, steamed not fried. White rice, if brown is not available. Order a baked potato with low-fat plain yogurt or whole wheat pasta without the sauce. If you desire sauce, request a Marinara over a cream sauce. Be warned however, some tomato based sauces are loaded with oils so ask how it is prepared.

For vegetables, request a salad with as many fresh colorful vegetables as possible and without cheeses or croutons. Order an olive oil based dressing on the side. If you're not shy, bring your own favorite dressing that is low in calories and fat. Or ask for a variety of vegetables to be steamed with no added butter or oils. For special occasions, have one glass of wine toward the end of the meal and pass on the dessert.

3. **If your meal isn't prepared as expected, send it back until they get it right.** If ordering a meal, for example egg white scramble and your eggs come back bright yellow with butter they used to fry it, send it back. I once had to do this three times until it was prepared the way I wanted it. The restaurants that get it right the first time deserve your repeat patronage. It's simply not worth sabotaging your healthy eating program because the chef has a different agenda.

4. **Do your research.** When deciding upon a restaurant, check out their website for nutrition information in advance. Select restaurants that not only are posting calories/protein/carbohydrates/fat, but are also providing healthy options.

5. **Stick to your favorite go-to restaurants.** Have your favorites available in times of dire need. Here's one of mine: Subway: Oven Roasted Chicken Sandwich. 6" on whole wheat, toasted and without cheese. Load up on the variety of vegetables and use mustard only, no mayo. Iced tea, no chips. Around 350 calories. Clean bathrooms a plus!

So You're Packing

Looking for a meal solution that is easy to take with you? Make healthy foods your new convenience food! A tool I've used over the years is to prepare my meals on the weekend, and keep them SIMPLE. A few healthy ingredients combined with a little pre-planning makes for nutritious meals that will keep you out of the fast-food lane.

The key is to prepare a nutritional balance of lean proteins, whole grains and vegetables in portable containers that you can keep in your refrigerator for days, if not a week and use them for your lunches or dinners.

325 Calorie On-The-Go Meal Template

Use this template for a single serving, and scale it up for as many meals as you would like to make, and would eat over the course of the work week. Switch out any of the lean meats, grains or vegetables for as much variety as possible.

- ✓ 1 ½ cups steamed or grilled veggies (as much variety as possible)
- ✓ ½ cup cooked grain brown rice, quinoa, barley or other whole grain
- ✓ 3 oz cooked grilled or broiled fish, spice-rubbed grilled chicken, shrimp or any other lean meat
- ✓ Any spice desired, go easy on the salt!
- ✓ Disposable containers such as Rubbermade TakeAlongs or equivalent

I tend to make about eight servings and store them in disposable containers, available at most grocery stores. Of course, I reuse them until they are no longer functional. I simply make the Quinoa, Brown Rice and Mushroom Medley—an original recipe in my book—or any whole grain in the rice cooker. While it's cooking, I steam the veggies and grill the meats—usually the Chicken Kabobs without the skewers—then partition equal portions in each container, then refrigerate. I often freeze them if it looks like I won't be able to eat them all within the week. Rice, incidentally, freezes quite well in freezer bags or containers.

Many options are available as far as totes are concerned. If you want to pack your lunch and look trendy and fabulous at the same time, go for an insulated tote instead of the brown bag (not so cute). The designs are fun, and if you feel sassy, go for a zebra print, or a contemporary design for a sophisticated look.

Just a little preparation goes a very long way. Experiment, have fun, and switch it up! It's a much healthier alternative than fast food or going hungry!

CHAPTER 14

PROGRESS REPORTS FROM
INSPIRATIONAL PEOPLE

*"Miracles happen every day, change your perception of what a
miracle is and you'll see them all around you."*

~Jon Bon Jovi

I wanted to share some inspirational stories with you about some of
my clients who I believe are remarkable; some even surprising and
miraculous! I wish I could include them all but I focused on the ones
who have fully embraced the concept of making incremental lifestyle
changes that are sustainable, and did not look upon this book as a
diet to be followed but an opportunity to start making better choices
for improved health, wellbeing, and quality of life. The photographs
are not labeled "before" and "after," because when it comes to lifestyle
changes there is no after, we are all ongoing work in progress. The
goal is to be as fit and healthy as possible throughout the many phases
of our lives. It is evident they started their journey in different places
and have made tremendous progress that will last them a lifetime;
maintaining their health when they encounter crisis, and making
progress as they can. Their ages range from their late 20s through
mid-60s and they demonstrate how it is never too late to raise your
personal wellness bar. If you think you can, you most certainly will
succeed.

Meet Richard and Heather

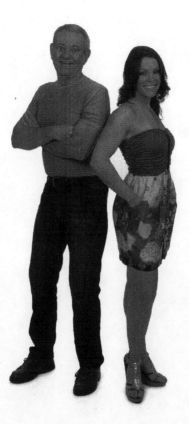

This photo of Heather, standing next to Richard, demonstrates the 130 pounds that she now weighs, equivalent to the amount of weight Richard lost. They both have not only lost the weight, but have made steady improvements since their initial loss for over one year!

Richard and Heather are co-workers, and as he began witnessing Heather's transformation he became curious as to what she was doing. Heather had begun her own journey and is an inspiration to everyone she knows. Richard had struggled for years with his weight, topping out at 315 pounds in his mid-sixties, with weight related health issues. I met with Richard one time for a lifestyle coaching session and listened to his story. He seemed frustrated and fatigued after regaining all 80 pounds from a failed high-protein diet, and was under the misconception that "carbs are bad for you." I explained to him how to make modifications to his eating regimen that are SUSTAINABLE; he purchased this book and went to work. He is most remarkable as he transitioned from a "diet" to a "lifestyle change" and within a year hit his goal of losing 130 pounds, down to a healthy 185 pounds, and most importantly is now off all his medications and has a renewed vitality—his skin simply glows.

Richard Morse—65, Fremont, CA

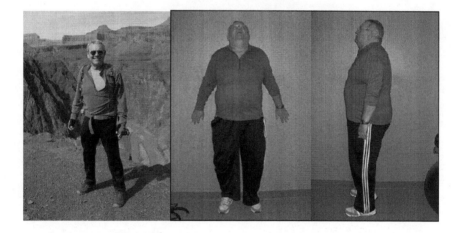

A few words from Richard: "You are what you eat," so eat healthy and clean. "BITE ME!" is more than a book of fantastic recipes; it is a book that will help you make a life style change to eating healthy clean foods that taste good and are good for you.

I began my lifestyle change at age 63 and a very unhealthy 315 lb. Initially I began using a low carbohydrate diet that was high in protein and fat. I was so out of shape that a 100 yard walk would have me out of breath, my hamstring muscles would burn. The low carbohydrate diet is not healthy or sustainable for long periods of time. After months on the low carbohydrate diet I lost weight but my body fat was a very unhealthy 31.3%.

I watched in disbelief as my good friend and coworker, Heather Buchholz continued to lose weight eating clean healthy foods from the BITE ME! book; fresh fruits, vegetables and interesting foods that I couldn't touch on my low carbohydrate diet. After months of toughing it out on the low carb diet eating food that tasted like particleboard, I was ready for a change in diet.

Heather introduced me to Toni and the BITE ME! book in November 2009. Toni asked me, "What is your daily calorie intake?" I had no idea; other than I was obviously burning more calories that I was consuming or I would not be losing weight. Toni encouraged me to get a calorie-monitoring armband so that I could monitor and determine the daily amount of calorie intake vs. the daily amount of calories burned. I got the armband and continue to use it daily.

I have lost 130 lb. and my body fat has been reduced to 24.7%. My blood pressure has been reduced from 120/80 to 103/58 and my total cholesterol has been reduced to 87 from 115, and I am completely off my blood pressure and cholesterol medications.

BITE ME! is not a fad diet that requires purchasing special foods from a single source; BITE ME! is a life style change that is sustainable because the foods taste good and the ingredients can be purchased from many high quality food suppliers. I don't leave home without my insulated cooler of BITE ME! Staples: Apple Carrot Bran Muffins, Apple Protein Bars, PB2. The BITE ME! Anti-Oxidant Three-Berry Protein Smoothie is a daily favorite and is my substitute for unhealthy ice cream.

Today I am in the best shape I have been since college, I walk or hike about 15 miles per week, I work out twice a week with a personal trainer and eat all my food from the Bite Me book. My goal is to reduce my weight to 190 lb. and body fat to under 20% (healthy for a 35 year old, great for a 65 year old). Get started with healthy life style by using the BITE ME! book and an exercise plan.

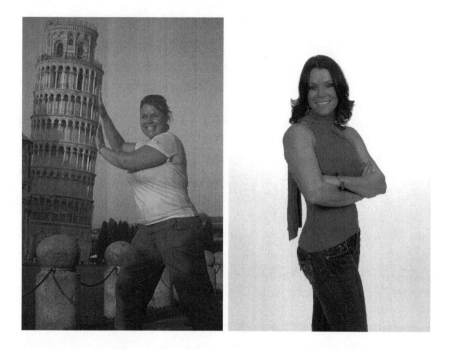

Heather Buchholz—30, San Jose, CA

When I was approached with the opportunity to do the BITE ME! Challenge—the BITE ME! eight week lifestyle change program—I was in a place in my life where I had already lost 65 pounds, but was struggling with the last ten or fifteen. Something had to give, I had exhausted all other options; literally from diet changes, or work out switch ups, I couldn't figure out how I couldn't get that ten off! I was ready for some drastic changes in my life and decided over the past 29 years I had put enough harmful things into my body that eight weeks of clean eating couldn't kill me but only make me stronger, literally.

When I embarked on this journey, we started off with an official body dunk, one of the most efficient and accurate ways to measure body fat percentage. I dunked starting out at 22% body fat, weighing in at 143. My end results were I ended up at 19% and weighed in at 130, and now I am at 14.9% body fat. That is an amazing transformation in itself alone, and numbers do not lie!

I thought I had eating dialed but I only had a portion of it down, which was portion control in itself. I had no clue what was behind clean eating. It consisted of pure, unprocessed, lean foods rich in nutrients and low in saturated fat. Exactly what my body needed; a shock! I ate solely out of this book for eight weeks solid. I gave up all alcohol and diet sodas. I gave this time to me, and turned all my focus to myself, and my health, because I am worth it.

This book and my determination have changed me for the better, for life. I will always incorporate these recipes and this style of eating in my life, and my future family's life. They will only know good, healthy nutrition and that inspires me. Since I have done this challenge I have had numerous people ask me, "What are doing, what is different, you are shrinking!" All I can do is forward them the link to this book, and smile because I know what lies behind the first turned page—a change to your life forever if you are ready to take that leap of faith! Cheers to your health!

Kara Jovalusky—42, San Jose, CA

Before I met Toni or heard about her program, I worked out three times a week with a personal trainer and went to kickboxing classes 2-3 times a week. However, after doing this consistently for almost a year it began to dawn on me that I was doing something wrong. I could not to lose any weight and all of that exhausting work seemed to be for nothing. Once Toni told me about her concept it became apparent why the weight would not come off: I was not eating properly. I was also working out way too much and not giving my body the materials it needed for proper recuperation. I began cooking from the recipes in her book, shortly thereafter, became a member of the Booty Club, their outdoor personalized training program. Not only did I finally begin to lose some of the weight that I had been trying so desperately to shed, I began to feel better and people tell me that I have never looked better in my life!

The only thing I hoped to achieve from this program was to lose some weight. However, I was pleasantly surprised by the fact that I also gained strength and muscle tone. As I began to cook from Toni's book, I learned how to cook food that was good for me and that tasted great. When I first started working out, I had my body fat measured. With my body fat at 31% and weighing in at 189 pounds, I started a workout and kickboxing routine. However, after that year of exhaustive effort, I still weighed about 185 pounds and was so frustrated that I did not even bother getting my body fat measured again. But after being on Toni's program for about six months, my body fat is down to 23.2 % and I now weigh 174 pounds. Wow, I've never felt better in my life! My husband, my family and all of my co-workers say that I look terrific! (I've gone from size 14 jeans down to a size 10). Now I know what cooking more healthy means and what foods I need to avoid and why. One benefit of her program is that I can now taste the fat in the foods that are not good for me to eat, which helps make it easier to avoid them. Her BITE ME! program has literally changed the way I feel about, look at and eat food.

Toni's motivation, sincerity, and her friendship have been a very important part of my success. She really does care about each and every one of those who come to her for help with their weight; and she proves that she cares by showing them how to eat properly and how to get in shape and stay fit. The other women I have met in the program have also become inspirations to me, as we all encourage each other to stick with the program and work hard to meet our goals. We are all there for one another; we lift each other up and help each other stay focused. This program has literally changed the way I look and feel about life and it has been a real game-changer for me. I heartily recommend this program for anyone who wants to learn about good nutrition, feeling great, losing weight and staying fit.

Chris Wagemann—47, San Jose, CA

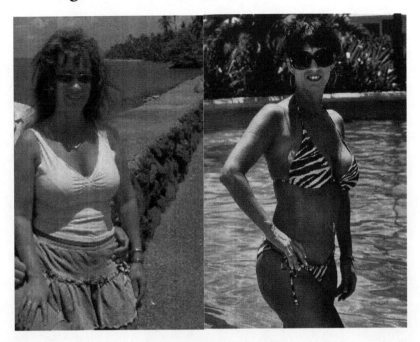

My weight loss journey started when I realized I weighed in at 148lbs and something had to give and fast. That was truly the heaviest I had ever weighed. I had nowhere else to turn, and I had heard many success stories from people who had joined Jenny Craig. I decided I would go for it! With that program I begin my journey and in its entirety I lost about 15 lbs. For someone of my height at 5"0 tall that is a HUGE loss, and I was excited, yet with the weighs-ins starting to stay the same, I wanted more! The summer came and went and my weight was going up and down. I then started an exercise class and my weight eventually hit a plateau again at 130, and I was still doing the Jenny Craig plan. I was now working out six times a week pretty religiously. I knew it wasn't my work out activity, so next to that it had to be my eating. One of the girls told us about a book called "BITE ME!" and brought a copy in to give some of us a tutorial of what it consisted of. She said it was clean eating and I had watched her shrink by eating out of this book first hand. I had her forward me the link. I checked it out and decided to purchase it and give it a try. This day completely changed my life and I haven't looked back since.

I started in early January weighing in at 129.6 lbs. It has been about two and half months so far and by eating out of this book I am proud to say I am currently at 116 pounds and I have lost many inches also. I have my high school waste line back; who wouldn't want that? I feel amazing and I look amazing. I am that get-up-and-go kind of woman now; nothing can hold me back. On top of looking good, I feel the best I have ever felt. My skin is glowing and radiant, and my clothes fit me the way I have always wanted them to.

I never thought I would lose these last 10 lbs. But with the right information and help from some friends, I have done it!

Laurina Lanham
Age 27, San Jose, CA

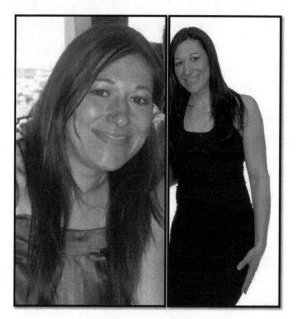

At the age of 27 I found myself in a place that I was not comfortable with but I had no idea how to get over the hurdles that plagued me. I consider myself an athlete; I ran track, played volleyball and remained active throughout high school and well into my college years. My health was never something I worried about, until this past year. I slowly noticed my health deteriorating and my body was failing me. I tried to work out on a daily basis but my body was no longer recovering as quickly as it once had and I developed so many aches and pains that the only place I found comfort was on the couch. I began to develop migraines and experienced once a week, sometimes once a day. I knew a change needed to be made; I was tired of being tired I was in dire need of a reality check. I relied too heavily on migraine pills that made me too drowsy to work out, and I found myself sleeping when I should have been living. I did not want to rely on medicine anymore when the real problem was my lifestyle. After looking in the mirror at myself, I realized that I was standing in my own way and it was vital that I do something to get my health back.

I was introduced to BITE ME! at a time where I could not have been more receptive to change. I studied this book, made my daily menus, did my shopping and cooked my food. A week into the book I started noticing a difference in my energy levels and I became much more aware of what I was putting into my body. I began paying attention to nutrition labels and what once seemed so foreign to me was suddenly clear. I soon realized that I was only paying attention to calories and Trans fat; I never thought to look at protein-to-carb ratio or saturated fat. I took inventory in my kitchen and threw out anything that did not fit the guidelines of the book; I did not want to be tempted. If I was going to do this for real I had to throw all excuses out and be honest with myself about what was really contributing to my health. By the second week of the book my friends and family began to notice a change, several people told m that my moods were better and they were right! I felt better and my attitude began to transform. I felt better in those first two weeks than I felt in the last year. I had the tools for taking back my health and I was stunned at the results.

My clean eating habits continue; this is not a diet, it's a lifestyle. I refer to the BITE ME! book on a daily basis. This was the change that needed to be made. Within the first week I did not have a single migraine; in fact I have not had a migraine since adapting the clean eating to my daily routine. As it turned out, prior to starting BITE ME!, my doctor informed me that the reason I was experiencing fatigue and migraines was due to a lack of sleep, anemia, and I was on my way to becoming pre-diabetic. It came as no surprise to me that after the eight weeks my fatigue turned to energy, and my migraines are non-existent. By taking on the principles of BITE ME! eating six small meals a day every two to three hours I was able to recharge my metabolism and retrain my body.

I am currently in the process of completing my graduate degree and I work full time, if I do not take care of my health and eat clean I will burn out. I know, because prior to finding this book I did exactly that. I cannot expect my body to perform at its best if I am not fueling it with the best. I was in need of a lifestyle makeover and this book did just that, it changed my life for good. All the unhealthy food I was putting into my body no longer appeals to me; I plan my meals out and remember the clean eating principles so that I can always make good decisions. I am in the best physical shape I have ever been in and I continue to push myself to the next level because I know that I can do it.

I truly believe that this book saved my health. I started it at 136 lbs, unhealthy and close being diagnosed as pre diabetic. I lost 30 pounds, four dress sizes and tested at 20% body fat; my health is the best it has ever been and the best part is that I made the change. With the tools in this book I was able to build a better life for myself and I could not be more grateful for the opportunity to be introduced to a wonderful group of women who continue to inspire and motivate me and I say "BITE ME!" to anyone who tries to pull me backwards. This book transformed me, and given the chance, it can do the same for you!

Debbie McCarrick-Olsen
Age 54, San Jose, CA

I have always been very conscious about eating right and exercise has been a top priority in my life. I was finding that my hard work was just not giving me the results I thought I should have, given all the hours

I logged in at the gym and constantly dieting. I decided to sign up with Adam (an unbelievable personal trainer) who was the caveat I needed to tweak things just enough to see and feel a difference. He in turn introduced me to Toni who had a big influence on my diet. It wasn't that I was eating poorly but the reaction of certain foods in my body were not allowing me to see positive results in fact I was working harder and gaining weight and feeling worse than ever. Being in my menopause years, I had sleepless nights and daytime and nighttime sweats or hot flashes—about one to two every hour. I had discussed hormone therapy with my doctor, which was a last resort.

Most importantly Toni really gave me a handle on my clean eating. I really boosted up the protein. I was eating more than ever but my choices were much different. No white bread, no white rice, no white potato. Instead I really kept an eye on my calories and all those hidden things we do from day to day, which really add up. I went to whole wheat, brown rice and sweet potato and learned about the benefits of fiber and flax seed. Since my passion is cooking I discovered great ways to cook fish and chicken. My refrigerator is stacked with veggies and fruit.

I went from 145 pounds and exercising five to six times per week to 130 exercising with the same exercise regimen. I have the occasional hot flash but am sleeping pretty much through the night. I am no longer feeling that bloated feeling and I am regular like clockwork—something that has never happened in my life.

Since I am Italian and grew up with pasta, bread and wine I think it is really important not to deprive yourself. I am cooking mostly with whole-wheat pasta. Occasionally if I eat the "old way" I quickly remember why I made new choices. Everything comes back like a freight train; 5 pounds just like that, no sleeping and a permanent fan attached to my head.

I am so grateful for the information given to me, and although I feel it is always a work in progress . . . learning new things about exercising and diet has really brought me to my "HAPPY PLACE."

Susan Lewis
Age 49, Pleasanton, CA

I was always a fat child, but never gave it much thought until I got a little older and had to shop in the "husky" department at Sears. I felt humiliated and that is probably when I first became aware that I was fat. I never really liked exercise and of course loved all things fattening, especially sweets. It was not until I was in the 7th grade that I began my relationship with dieting. I had been asked to be in my Aunt's wedding, and in order to be a junior brides-maid, I had to fit into a borrowed size 5 dress. I decided to start to count my calories and limit myself to 1000 calories a day. I wrote down everything I ate and stuck to my 1000 calories diligently. Some days that would mean I ate a Snickers bar, 5 Oreos and ice cream, but it was still 1000 calories and I fit into the dress. So, needless to say, I stuck with that method for a long time . . . like 30 years! When I got pregnant, I knew I had to eat healthier and found I worried less about calories, a little and more about nutrition, but once the baby was born, I was right back to my old habits and that is pretty much how I have maintained my weight my whole life. As I begin to age and get a little wiser, I have gotten more concerned about my overall health, but still want to be slender and fit.

About two years ago, I met Toni at a party and was attracted to her immediately. She looked how I would like to look and I was so curious to find out how she did it. We spoke a lot about eating and exercise habits and what I loved about her instantly is she was a genuine person and had some of the same struggles I did. She suggested I keep a food log for three days and then send her what I ate . . . an honest account. That was a little challenging because I was embarrassed to send her what my honest account was, but I wanted to make some changes, so felt I needed to start there.

She was super supportive and did not criticize, but instead told me how I could make little changes to improve. She suggested the body bug program to log my food, which also broke down the nutrients I needed so I could see where I was deficient. Toni made me much more aware of how important it is to make nutritional choices that really make a difference in the way you feel. I find I am much more aware of balancing proteins and adding more fruits and veggies to my diet and I find I can actually eat more. I have also been so motivated by the changes I've seen in my body and my energy levels that I have increased by exercise, which motivates me to eat better, which motivates me to exercise more and helps to create a more positive cycle of wellness overall. I still have a sweet tooth and definitely slip up every once in a while, but now I notice that I really don't feel good when I do that and get excited about feeling healthy. It is definitely worth it.

Victoria Pearce-Kelso
Age 50, San Jose, CA

When I started Toni's Booty Club four months ago, I was turning 50, was 40 pounds overweight and sedentary. I have anxiety and depression issues, which were getting worse. I had not worked out for about five years, and could not seem to find the will power or commitment to do it.

The first day was exciting but tough, they were genuinely interested in understanding me and what my issues were; they helped me adjust the workout to meet my ability level. I was the slowest and least in shape person there, but it did not seem to matter. Everyone was encouraging me, including the other members in the class. I needed a support system, people to count on me, and professionals to map out my work out. I noticed right away that my strength had increased; simple things like getting out of a deep chair and bending over were becoming easy. I had no idea how much I wasn't able to do until I started doing them again.

My energy and self-esteem increased. The depression and anxiety has decreased significantly. I lost 10 pounds without even changing my diet and inches started to come off, my fat layer was starting to disappear. Recently I started to eat healthy and dropped five more pounds in two weeks. I feel so much better; I never want to go back to the way I felt before. The Booty Club is always different; I never know what to expect so the time flies by. I don't know how they do it but the work out hits every part of my body, while increasing my stamina. Booty Club is truly an amazing work out and it's FUN! Without the supportive team I would have given up long ago! It would have been impossible for me to get this overall work out at the gym. Booty Club has changed my life!

Update: Victoria joined the BITE ME! Challenge recently and lost an additional 12 pounds in eight weeks through eating clean. Since joining the Booty Club, she has reduced her overall body fat by 18% in a seven month period, a tremendous accomplishment!

Peter Pravettoni
Age 52, Lewisville, Texas

I started with Toni in July of 2008 I weighed 232 lbs, my cholesterol and Triglycerides were very high and I was border-line diabetic. With advice from Toni on clean eating and a workout routine to fit my age and physical limitations I was able to lose 30 lbs in four months and to the surprise of my doctor my blood work was all excellent. Toni took care and paid constant attention to my workouts and nutritional intake on a daily basis. We did this almost exclusively over the Internet with a few phone calls here and there. I am a musician and need to be on stage and look, feel, and perform at a high level and this system has helped me to achieve my goals; I would recommend this to anyone.

CHAPTER 15

Ready, Get Set, Let's Eat!

Are you as excited as I am? You have a world of delicious eating ahead of you! I encourage you to go through the meal solutions and see what appeals to your palette. Feel free to experiment and swap some of the ingredients for some of your favorites. For example, if you love the Southern Greens Gone Clean recipe, but you prefer spinach and kale over the other greens, swap it out! Just be sure to keep it within the food groups. Don't eliminate a vegetable for a glass of wine or chunk of butter. You get the point!

Now some specialty items can be difficult to find if you haven't purchased them before. The majority of the ingredients you will find at your standard grocery store. Others, such as oat flour can be purchased at Whole Foods or online. You'll see abbreviations in parenthesis after the ingredient for these particular items. A little extra effort initially will go a long way in expanding your culinary horizons.

Even though the meal solutions and recipes are categorized into groups, they are listed in a way that is familiar to most people however you can feel free to enjoy any dish any time of the day. Enjoy!

UNDERSTANDING THE NUTRIENT PROFILE

Every recipe features a nutrient profile under the headline to make it easy to fully understand what you are consuming before you start cooking. It will look like this:

NUTRIENT PROFILE   CAL-178/PRO-8/CARB-30/FAT-4/SAT-0/
                                      CHO-300/SOD-58/FIB-6

PERCENT CALORIES FROM   PRO-17%/CARB-64%/FAT-19%

CAL=Calories
PRO=Protein
CARB=Carbohydrates
FAT=Total Fat (including Saturated Fat)
SAT=Saturated Fat
CHO=Cholesterol
SOD=Sodium
FIB=Fiber

PERCENT CALORIES FROM: Percentages are shown for protein, carbohydrates and fat for each serving. Because calories per gram vary by the nutrient—for example protein and carbohydrates are 4 calories per gram, alcohol is 7 and fat is a densely packed 9 calories per gram—these numbers indicate the percentage of the calories eaten for that meal. For example, in the Nutrition Profile, the recipe contains three grams of unsaturated fat. Multiplied by 9, the total amount of calories from fat is 27 out of 192 total calories, or 17%.

NUTRIENT DESCRIPTIONS:

Calories: Total calories per serving. To ensure accuracy when measuring your serving size, especially in the case of a large pot of soup, divide the meal in half, then divide equally until servings are individually portioned.

Protein: Proteins are essential for building and maintaining muscle mass. Neither fat nor carbohydrates can perform this function. Extra protein can be used as energy if there is an excess, however carbohydrates cannot perform this dual purpose. Individual protein requirements vary. To calculate your specific needs, the US RDA recommends .8 grams of protein per kilogram of bodyweight per day for the average person or between 15-30% of total calories. A bodybuilder or professional athlete recommended intake is 1.2 to 2.0 g/kg per day.

To calculate:
Convert your bodyweight in pounds, to kilograms
1 lb = .45359 kg
Example: 132 lbs x .45359 = 58.9 kg
58.9 kg x 1.2 = 70.68 grams of protein per day

Carbohydrates: Carbohydrates are necessary for brain function and energy. 50-70% of your total calories should come from carbohydrates. Complex carbohydrates are more slowly absorbed—as compared to simple carbohydrates—and create less of a blood sugar spike.

Total Fat: According to the US RDA, between 20-30% of calories can come from fat. The goal is to consume ZERO trans-fats and saturated fats. As a rule of thumb, try to keep total fat to 1 gram fat per 50 calories. For example the Nutrient Profile below illustrates total fat at 3 grams for 192 calories. 3-4 grams would be a reasonable amount of unsaturated, healthy fat for this meal, weighing in at 17% of the total calories. Most of the recipes are on the low end of the spectrum, around 15-20% although it varies. These percentages are taken from the quantity of calories that come from each of these sources. Be sure to consume healthy, unsaturated fats through supplementing your diet with olive oils and raw nuts and seeds, approximately three tablespoons each day.

Saturated Fat: All recipes in this book are very low in saturated fats and are often nonexistent in most. Saturated fats are primarily animal fats, such as fatty beef, bacon, cheese and butter, and should be kept to a minimum.

Unsaturated and polyunsaturated fats, such as Omega-3 are essential fats that your body needs to function properly but does not make. We must get them from food, such as salmon, tuna, sardines, mackerel or shellfish. Other essential oils include walnuts, flaxseed, and canola and soybean oils.

Cholesterol: This is the artery clogging type of fat; the less, the better.

Sodium: The RDA is 2400 mg per day. Be sure to read labels when buying canned, processed and even frozen foods, they can contain high levels sodium.

Fiber: The recommended fiber intake for adults is about 25 grams per day. Try the Antioxidant Protein Smoothie; it packs a powerful fiber punch in a single serving!

"A dream is just a dream. A goal is a dream with a plan and a deadline."

Recipes And Meal Solutions

USER FRIENDLY TIPS:

What's that and where do I get it? Some items may feel like they are hard to find, but not if you know where to look! So we've included icons on the most perplexing. (TJS) Trader Joe's (C) Costco (WF) Whole Foods (G) General Store (BO) Bob's Red Mill www.bobsredmill.com (BP) Bell Plantation www.bellplantation.com

Measuring Abbreviations
C = Cup ~ T = Tablespoon ~ t = Teaspoon

Jumpstart Your Day

BITE ME! Pumpkin Spice Steel Cut Oats

Makes 8 Servings

NUTRITION PROFILE   CAL-178/PRO-8/CARB-30/FAT-4/SAT-0/
                                       CHO-300/SOD-58/FIB-6

PERCENT CALORIES FROM   PRO-17%/CARB-64%/FAT-19%

Nothing hits the spot like a bowl of steel-cut oats in the morning. The best part of this dish is that you can make it once and it lasts for the week. Oat meal reheats to its original texture and the pumpkin spices meld beautifully.

Ingredients:

5 C	Boiling Water
1/2 t	Salt
2 C	Bob's Red Mill Organic Whole Grain Steel Cut Oats
1 1/3 C	Canned Pumpkin
4	Egg Whites
2 T	Flaxseed Meal
1 T	Cinnamon
1/2 t	Nutmeg
1 t	Ground Ginger
1/4 t	Ground Cloves
1/4 C	Agave Nectar (or honey)
4 T	Raw Pumpkin Seeds, Sunflower Seeds or Walnuts
4 T	Dried Cranberries

Per Serving: 2 t Nuts and Seeds
                   2 t Dried Cranberries

Instructions:

In medium saucepan with lid, combine salt and 5 cups water. Bring to boil. Stir in oats and reduce heat to low. Cook covered stirring occasionally.

In separate bowl, lightly whisk eggs and pumpkin mixture. Add all spices. Mix thoroughly.

Combine pumpkin mixture into cooked oats and stir, heating through for a couple of minutes. Put on warm setting. Add honey and stir through.

Pour into casserole or flat pan. Top with nuts, seeds and cranberries, and refrigerate up to one week. Once congealed, cut into eight servings. Delicious when reheated in microwave. Really!

Apple-Cinnamon Multi-Grain Oatmeal

Makes 8 Servings

NUTRITION PROFILE   CAL-178/PRO-8/CARB-30/FAT-4/SAT-0/
                     CHO-300/SOD-58/FIB-6

PERCENT CALORIES FROM   PRO-17%/CARB-64%/FAT-19%

Ingredients:

5 C	Boiling Water
½ t	Salt
3 C	Choice Organic Multi-Grain Hot Cereal (or Quaker Oats) (TJS)
3	Egg Whites
1 C	Unsweetened Applesauce
1	Chopped Apple, unpeeled
1 T	Flaxseed Meal
1 T	Cinnamon
½ t	Nutmeg
1 t	Ground Ginger
¼ C	Agave Nectar (or honey)
4 T	Raisins

Instructions:

In medium saucepan with lid, combine salt and 5 cups water. Bring to boil. Stir in grains and reduce heat to low. Cook covered stirring occasionally. Add apples, raisins and spices and allow to simmer for two minutes.

Combine applesauce and egg whites, mix well. Combine with cooked grain mixture and stir, heating through for a couple of minutes. Finally, mix honey into the mixture.

Pour into casserole or flat pan and refrigerate up to one week. Once congealed, cut into eight servings. Delicious when reheated in microwave.

Frittata Firenze

Makes 6 Servings

This recipe was born out of a love for all foods Italian as well as the desire for rich, cheesy flavors without the added calories. No one can tell there is cottage cheese in this dish as it is a delicate enhancement. Blending it into the egg mixture gives it a smooth, light texture and delicately balanced flavor. When combined with the Italian savory flavors of the olives, basil and tomato it is a true pleasure for the palette! For a nutritionally balanced meal, serve with fresh orange rounds and 100% whole wheat toast (included in the Nutrition Profile below).

NUTRITION PROFILE	CAL-240/PRO-17/CARB-35/FAT-4/SAT-1/
	CHO-3/SOD-649/FIB-9
PERCENT CALORIES FROM	PRO-27%/CARB-57%/FAT-16%

Ingredients:

12	Egg Whites plus 2 Egg Yolks
1/3 c	Low Salt Chicken Broth
¾ c	Low fat Cottage Cheese 1%
2 c	Fresh Spinach
1	Yellow Onion, chopped
1 Jar	Artichoke Hearts (in water)
¼ c	Kalamata Olives, chopped
2 T	Shredded or Grated Romano Cheese
1 c	Fresh Mushrooms
1 t	Garlic Powder
2 t	chopped Fresh Basil or substitute 1 t Dried
1 t	Ground Cayenne Red Pepper
1 T	Kirkland Brand Organic No Salt Seasoning or substitute Onion and Garlic Power

½ t	Salt or to taste
½ t	White or Black Pepper
¼ c	Tomato Sauce
1 t	Olive Oil, or Olive Oil cooking spray

| 6 | Fresh Oranges (cut into round slices) |
| 6 | Whole Wheat Toast |

Instructions:

Sautee mushrooms and onions using olive oil or nonstick cooking spray. In blender, combine chicken broth, eggs and nonfat cottage cheese, along with all dry spices and blend until creamy and smooth.
In round Pyrex baking dish, layer spinach, olives, mushroom, and onion mixture. Pour egg mixture over layered vegetables in dish. To garnish arrange thinly sliced tomatoes and spinach leaves on top. For holidays, garnish with three fresh basil or spinach leaves in a holly arrangement with three olive halves for the berries.

Bake at 350 for 45 minutes. Brush top around garnish with tomato sauce and return to oven about 20 minutes.

Peanut Butter Yogurt Crunch! Parfait

Makes 1 Serving

NUTRITION PROFILE	CAL-305/PRO-25/CARB-46/FAT-4/SAT-0/
	CHO-7/SOD-278/FIB-4
PERCENT CALORIES FROM	PRO-31%/CARB-57%/FAT-12%

Ingredients:

2 T   PB2
½ c   Nonfat Vanilla Yogurt
½ c   GoLEAN Crunch! Cereal
¼ c   Fresh Blueberries and Raspberries

Instructions:

Mix PB2 and vanilla yogurt. Layer ½ of the yogurt mixture in bottom of a clear glass or bowl. Top with ¼ c of cereal, then the remaining yogurt, cereal and berries to top.

Chocolate Peanut Butter French Toast

Makes 1 Serving

NUTRITION PROFILE   CAL-329/PRO-29/CARB-45/FAT-5/SAT-1/
                        CHO-0/SOD-246/FIB-7
PERCENT CALORIES FROM   PRO-34%/CARB-53%/FAT-13%

Ingredients:
2   Egg Whites or equivalent
1 t   Vanilla
2   Slices Orowheat 100% Whole Wheat Bread

Topping:
½ t   Cocoa Powder
2 T   PB2 (find at www.bellplantation.com)
½ c   Greek Strained Yogurt or Nonfat Plain Yogurt

Instructions:
Mix egg whites with vanilla in bowl. Dip both sides of the bread and cook in pan until browned, turning once. Mix yogurt, cocoa powder and PB2. Top French toast and enjoy!

Greek strained yogurt is delicious. It's slightly tarter than other nonfat plain yogurts. The best price found by far is at Trader Joe's.

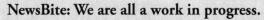

NewsBite: We are all a work in progress.
Make changes one at a time, changes you can live with. Once that is mastered, make another one. The more you change, the better you will feel; which will encourage you to make more positive changes. Above all, be kind to yourself. If you make a poor eating choice, your next bite can be a healthy one!

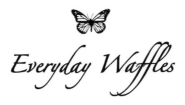

Everyday Waffles

Makes 4 Servings

NUTRITION PROFILE   CAL-199/PRO-21/CARB-19/FAT-4/SAT-0/
                                      CHO-7/SOD-94/FIB-2
PERCENT CALORIES FROM   PRO-42%/CARB-39%/FAT-19%

Ingredients:

3	Egg Whites
2 t	Olive Oil
1 ½ c	Nonfat Milk
½ c	Whole Wheat Flour
½ c	Oat Flour
2/3 c	Met Rx Protein Powder (Vanilla Flavor)
¼ t	Salt
½ t	Baking Powder

For Chocolate waffles, add 1 Tablespoon unsweetened cocoa powder and use chocolate flavored Met Rx!

Instructions:

Whisk egg whites in bowl. Add milk and olive oil and stir, and then set aside. In separate bowl, mix flours, protein powder, cocoa, salt and baking powder. Combine wet and dry ingredients by hand until blended.

Spray waffle iron with non-stick spray coating. On medium high setting, use approximately ¼ of the batter to make each waffle. Cook until browned and slightly crispy.

Serving Suggestion: Top with nonfat yogurt mixed with PB2!

Time Saving Tip: Double the batch and freeze for future meals. To re-warm, toast until crispy and heated through.

Take With You Treats

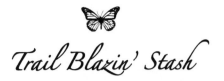

Trail Blazin' Stash

Makes 6 Servings (1/2 cup each)

When my supply of available fresh snacks is depleted, I keep my special stash on hand. Contrary to popular belief, not all fats have a negative impact. Nuts and seeds are an important part of one's diet, although because they are so calorie dense they should be eaten in moderation. Always portion your servings into small baggies rather than just grabbing a handful. Raw nuts are ideal. Roasted nuts are delicious as long as no added oils or salts are used.

NUTRITION PROFILE	CAL-194/PRO-5/CARB-20/FAT-12/SAT-1/
	CHO-0/SOD-2/FIB-3
PERCENT CALORIES FROM	PRO-9%/CARB-39%/FAT-52%

Ingredients:

1/2 c   Raw Sunflower Seeds
1 c   Freeze Dried Banana Slices (TJS)
1/2 c   (about 10) Unsweetened Apple Rings, chopped (TJS)
1/2 c   Raw Walnuts (C)
1/2 c   Raisins (C)

Instructions:

Place all ingredients into bowl. Divide into five, ½ cup portions and place in baggies for a quick on the go snack.

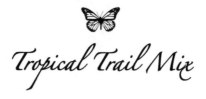

Tropical Trail Mix

Makes 5 servings (1/2 cup each)

This particular blend is my favorite. Dried fruit is often processed with added sugars which not only add unwanted, empty calories to your snack but spike your blood sugar. Stick with natural dried fruits and read the ingredients label!

NUTRITION PROFILE   CAL-224/PRO-12/CARB-32/FAT-17/SAT-1/
                           CHO-15/SOD-25/FIB-7
PERCENT CALORIES FROM   PRO-14%/CARB-39%/FAT-47%

Ingredients:

1/2 c   Dried Mango (WF)
1/2 c   Dried Blueberries
½ c   Dried Cranberries (C)
1/2 c   Raw Almonds (C)
1/2 c   Raw Pepitos (pumpkin seeds) (TJS)

Instructions:

Place all ingredients into bowl. Divide into five, ½ cup portions and place in baggies for a quick on the go snack.

Toni's Protein-Berry Mini-Bundt's

Makes 18 muffins or 24 mini-bundt cakes
Serving Size: One mini-bundt (the regular muffin size is approx 150 calories)

Each bite offers a burst of juicy berries. It's seems like an indulgence but it's not, it's clean and healthy. I use a variety of protein powders and always look for the words "protein concentrate" first in the ingredients list. Secondly, I look for the highest protein to lowest fat ratio. You can use pure "whey" which is better absorbed over soy protein.

NUTRITION PROFILE	CAL-103/PRO-9/CARB-12/FAT-3/SAT-0/ CHO-2/SOD-83/FIB-2
PERCENT CALORIES FROM	PRO-34%/CARB-45%/FAT-21%

Ingredients:

1 c	Egg Whites
1 ½ c	Oats
1 c	Nonfat Cottage Cheese (or substitute nonfat plain yogurt)
1 c	Nonfat Milk
1 c	Unsweetened Applesauce
1 T	Vanilla Extract
1 C	Whole Wheat Flour
½ C	Oat Bran (TJS)
1 ½ C	Whey Protein Powder—Vanilla
1 ½ t	Baking Powder
1 ½ t	Baking Soda
1/8 t	Salt
25	Almonds or ½ C Walnuts
2 C	Three Berries (Frozen Raspberries, Blueberries and Marion berries—Available at Costco) or Substitute Fresh

Instructions:

Pre-heat oven to 350 degrees. First, defrost frozen berries for approximately six minutes in microwave and set aside. Pour egg whites, oats and cottage cheese into blender and blend on low until smooth. Combine all ingredients (except for the berries) into mixing bowl and mix on medium until blended. Fold in fruit (un-drained) by hand to retain the integrity of the berries. Spray mini-bunt or muffin tins with non-stick cooking spray. Because bundts are upside down in the pan, sprinkle a few raw oats, and a scant amount of brown sugar in the bottom of each cup. Fill 2/3's full with batter. Bake at 350 for 20 minutes. Allow to sit about five minutes and flip them out onto a towel. Cool on wire rack.

Time Saving Tip: With the perfect blend of protein, carbohydrates and healthy fats, these bundts make a delicious and easy breakfast or on the go snack. Freeze them in baggies of two each so you'll always have them on hand.

Apple Carrot Bran Muffins

Makes 18 Servings

NUTRITION PROFILE   CAL-141/PRO-10/CARB-21/FAT-6/SAT-0/
                           CHO-2/SOD-35/FIB-5
PERCENT CALORIES FROM   PRO-22%/CARB-46%/FAT-32%

Ingredients:

1 ¼ c	Whole Wheat Flour
¾ c	Flaxseed Meal
¾ c	Oat Bran
1 c	Whey Protein (3 scoops Vanilla Protein Powder)
½ c	Turbinado or Washed Raw Natural Sugar
2 t	Baking Soda
1 t	Baking Powder
½ t	Salt
4 T	Cinnamon
1 ½ c	Carrots, Shredded
2	Apples, Peeled and Chopped, Including Skin
¾ c	Nonfat Milk
½ c	Egg Whites
1 tsp	Vanilla
½ c	Raw Almonds, chopped
2/3 c	Dried Cranberries

Instructions:

Mix all ingredients; fill baking cups to 2/3's full. Bake at 350 for 30 minutes, checking to make sure the toothpick comes out dry. It's the perfect ratio of protein to carbohydrates to healthy fats needed at each meal.

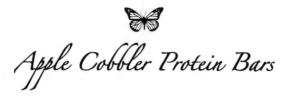

Apple Cobbler Protein Bars

Makes 12 Bars
Serving Size: 1 Bar

NUTRITION PROFILE   CAL-192/PRO-15/CARB-26/FAT-3/SAT-0/
                                 CHO-6/SOD-57/FIB-3
PERCENT CALORIES FROM   PRO-30%/CARB-53%/FAT-17%

Ingredients:

1 c	Oat Flour (WF) (B)
1 c	Whole Wheat Flour
1 1/3 c	Vanilla Whey Protein Powder
1 1/3 c	Nonfat Plain Yogurt
2	Large Egg Whites
1 c	Oat Bran
1 c	Turbinado, or Natural Raw Sugar (WF) (TJ)
1 c	Unsweetened Applesauce
3 TBS	Honey or Agave Nectar
1 Large	Apple, Chopped (don't peel)
4 T	Vanilla Extract
4 T	Cinnamon (or more if you dare!)
½ TSP	Salt
2 t	Baking Soda
2 T	Olive Oil

Instructions:

Preheat oven to 350 degrees. Combine in a large bowl: oat flour, whole wheat flour, salt, 2 TBS cinnamon and most of the Turbinado, reserving a couple of tablespoons for later. Stir dry ingredients together.

Mix the yogurt, egg whites, vanilla extract and olive oil until combined. Add the protein powder one scoop at a time, until thoroughly blended. Pour this mixture into the bowl of dry ingredients and stir together until it has the consistency of dough.

Coat an 8x12 inch baking pan with cooking spray, then flatten the dough into the pan, smoothing it up to the edges. Next, mix the applesauce, 2 T cinnamon, chopped apple and honey together and pour over the top of the dough mixture in the pan, spreading evenly. Sprinkle the oat bran over the top, until thoroughly and evenly covered, then sprinkle the remaining brown sugar over the top.

Bake for 30 minutes at 350 degrees. Switch to broil just until top is slightly browned, being careful not to overcook.

Bite Me! Banana Bread

Makes 8 Servings or 12 Muffins
Serving Size: 1/8 loaf

NUTRITION PROFILE   CAL-248/PRO-13/CARB-44/FAT-3/SAT-0/
                         CHO-3/SOD-44/FIB-5
PERCENT CALORIES FROM   PRO-20%/CARB-68%/FAT-27%

Ingredients:

Combine in a large bowl:
1 c   Whole Wheat Flour
1 c   Oat Flour (WF) (B)
2/3 c   Vanilla Protein Powder
1/2 t   Salt
1/2 t   Baking Soda
1 t   Baking Powder

Combine separately:

2   Egg Whites
5 T   Agave Nectar (or honey)
1/2 c   Nonfat Milk
1 T   Zest of an Orange, coarsely grated
½ c   Unsweetened Applesauce
2 T   Bacardi Limon Rum, Limón cello or 2 ts Vanilla Extract
1/4 c   Chopped Walnuts or Almonds

Add Last: 1 ¾ c Ripe Bananas, mashed (about 3 large)

Instructions:

Using a mixer, combine dry ingredients and set aside. Combine wet ingredients and add to the dry, except the banana, just until incorporated. Fold in banana and stir by hand so the chunks of fruit are retained. It creates a moist and better textured muffin. Pour into a nonstick loaf pan sprayed with nonstick cooking spray. Bake at 350 for about 50 min—a toothpick inserted in center should come out clean. Wait 10 minutes before removing from pan and place on a rack to cool. Cut into 8 slices.

For an On-The-Go option, make 12 muffins. Each muffin 165 calories, 9 grams of protein, 29 carbohydrates and only 2 grams of fat. Garnish with 3 small pieces of chopped walnuts each. Bake at 350 for 20 minutes.

Purely Pumpkin Muffins

Makes 18 Muffins
Serving Size: 1 Muffin

NUTRITION PROFILE   CAL-114/PRO-10/CARB-15/FAT-2/SAT-0/
                        CHO-4/SOD-90/FIB-2
PERCENT CALORIES FROM   PRO-36%/CARB-51%/FAT-13%

(Tip: buy the canned pumpkin in the winter months and save it, it's a seasonal item)

Combine in large bowl:

1 c	Whole Wheat Flour
1 c	Oat Flour (WF)
2/3 c	Vanilla Protein Powder
½ t	Salt
½ t	Baking Soda
1 t	Baking Powder
1 T	Cinnamon
1 T	Pumpkin Pie Spice
½ t	Ground Cloves

Combine separately:

1 T	Olive Oil
2	Egg Whites
½ c	Rice Dream or Non-Fat Milk
1 c	Canned Pumpkin (G) Seasonal Item

½ c   Unsweetened Applesauce
2 T   Triple Sec
3 T   Honey or Agave Nectar

Instructions:

Using a mixer, combine wet and dry ingredients, just until incorporated. Spoon into muffin tins. Bake at 350 for about 25 minutes.

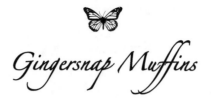

Gingersnap Muffins

12 Muffins
Serving Size: 1 Muffin

NUTRITION PROFILE   CAL-152/PRO-16/CARB-22/FAT-2/SAT-0/
                                   CHO-6/SOD-45/FIB-3
PERCENT CALORIES FROM   PRO-38%/CARB-50%/FAT-12%

Ingredients:

1 c	Whole Wheat Flour
1 c	Oat Flour (WF)
2/3 c	Vanilla Protein Powder
1/2 tsp	Salt
1 T	Ground Ginger
1 t	Allspice
1 t	Ground Pepper
1 t	Baking Soda
1 t	Baking Powder
3	Egg Whites
3 T	Agave Nectar (or honey)
2 T	Molasses (Brer Rabbit All Natural Molasses)
1/2 c	Nonfat Milk
1 T	Olive Oil
1 c	Unsweetened Applesauce

Instructions:

Using a mixer, combine dry ingredients, mix in wet until just until incorporated. Spoon into muffin tins. Bake at 350 for about 25 minutes.

Apricot Molasses Bran Muffins

Makes 12 Muffins
Serving Size: 1 Muffin

NUTRITION PROFILE	CAL-158/PRO-9/CARB-29/FAT-2/SAT-0/CHO-2/SOD-41/FIB-4
PERCENT CALORIES FROM	PRO-21%/CARB-67%/FAT-12%

Ingredients:

1 c	Whole Wheat Flour
1 c	Kellogs All-Bran BranBuds (G)
1 c	Oat Flour (WF) (B)
2/3 c	Vanilla Protein Powder
1/2 tsp	Salt
1 t	Baking Soda
1 t	Baking Powder
3	Egg Whites
3 T	Agave Nectar (or honey)
2 T	Molasses (Brer Rabbit All Natural Molasses)
1 1/2 c	Nonfat Milk
1 T	Canola or Olive Oil
1 c	Unsweetened Applesauce
½ c	Chopped Dried Apricots

Instructions:

In small bowl, combine 1 cup of the milk and the Bran Buds. Set aside and allow to soften while combining the remaining ingredients. Using a mixer, combine all ingredients and mix until smooth. Add the remaining ½ c milk and mix until incorporated. Pour into a nonstick

161

muffin pan sprayed with Pam or equivalent. Top with a few small apricot pieces on each muffin and bake at 350 for about 25 min—a toothpick inserted in center should come out clean. Wait 10 minutes before removing from pan and place on a rack to cool.

NewsBite: Make your muffins pop!

Because the muffin recipes in this book have no added fat, they can be more challenging to remove from the pans, but don't let that deter you! Unless you like eating bits of paper, avoid the paper muffin cups completely. Spray your muffin tins directly with Pam or use a paper towel or cotton ball and lightly moisten tins with Grape seed Oil, then add a dusting of oat flour. After baking, allow the muffins to cool about 10 minutes. Use a bamboo skewer to loosen around the edges of each muffin. It won't scratch and works much better than a butter knife. Give the muffin a quick turn, and pop it out! Yum . . . . hot muffins!

The Guiltless PB² & J Sandwich

Makes 1 Serving

NUTRITION PROFILE	CAL-260/PRO-14/CARB-40/FAT-6/SAT-1/
	CHO-0/SOD-244/FIB-7
PERCENT CALORIES FROM	PRO-19%/CARB-58%/FAT-23%

Such a simple recipe, yet SO delicious! It's truly a guilt free indulgence and for those days when you've already eaten your healthy raw nuts. This recipe calls for PB2. If you are a peanut butter lover, PB2 is 85% LESS FAT. It's cold pressed, similar to the process of making extra virgin olive oil, except they lose the oil and keep all the pea nutty goodness. The consistency is not quite as smooth as original peanut butter, primarily because it has less fat, and comes in a powder form so it can be reconstituted. But in this sandwich, you won't know the difference. After a figure competition, it's the first food I crave, and for extra crunchy texture, I add a small amount of chopped peanuts (included in the Nutrient Profile). Although this appeals to kids, I sometimes will take a cookie cutter and cut a special shape in the middle. It just makes me feel eight years old again!

You can find PB2 online at *www.bellplantation.com*

Ingredients:

2 T	PB2 (un-constituted) (BP)
1 T	Apricot Simply Fruit Jam
1 T	Coarsely Chopped Peanuts
2 Slices	100% Whole Wheat or Ezekiel Bread, toasted

Instructions:

Mix PB2 with 1 T water. Spread to one piece of whole wheat toast. Apply the Apricot Jam to the other piece of toast. Sprinkle with chopped peanuts and assemble.

Booty Kickin' Boosts

Chocolate-Banana Smoothie

Makes 1 Smoothie

NUTRITION PROFILE	CAL-290/PRO-36/CARB-20/FAT-4/SAT-1/ CHO-13/SOD-153/FIB-2
PERCENT CALORIES FROM	PRO-48%/CARB-40%/FAT-12%

Ingredients:

1 T	Cocoa powder
1/3 c	(1 scoop) Chocolate Protein Powder
1 cup	Nonfat Milk
1	Ripe Banana (can be frozen or fresh)
2 t	Agave Nectar

Blend with ice cubes in blender, a few at a time, for desired consistency.

Time Saving Tip: Take your ripe bananas and puree them, then freeze them in ice cube trays. You won't need to add ice and you'll always have bananas on hand!

Coffee Chocolate-Mint Protein Smoothie

Makes 1 Smoothie

NUTRITION PROFILE   CAL-225/PRO-30/CARB-25/FAT-1/SAT-0/
                           CHO-13/SOD-18/FIB-2
PERCENT CALORIES FROM   PRO-54%/CARB-44%/FAT-2%

Ingredients:

¾ c   Nonfat Milk
¾ c   Decaf Coffee
2 T   Cocoa Powder
1/3 c   (1 scoop) Chocolate Protein Powder
3 Drops   Mint Extract
2 t   Agave Nectar

Instructions:

Blend with about nine ice cubes in blender, add more or less for desired consistency.

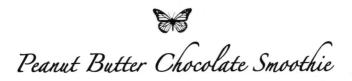

Peanut Butter Chocolate Smoothie

Makes 1 Smoothie

NUTRITION PROFILE	CAL-311/PRO-38/CARB-31/FAT-5/SAT-1/
	CHO-12/SOD-199/FIB-1
PERCENT CALORIES FROM	PRO-48%/CARB-38%/FAT-14%

Ingredients:

2 T   PB2
1 T   Cocoa powder
1/3 c   (1 scoop) Chocolate Protein Powder
1 cup   Nonfat Milk
2 t   Agave Nectar or Honey

Instructions:

Blend with ice cubes, a few at a time, in blender for desired consistency.

Antioxidant Protein Smoothie

Makes 1 Serving

NUTRITION PROFILE   CAL-351/PRO-39/CARB-34/FAT-13/SAT-1/
                            CHO-13/SOD-73/FIB-10
PERCENT CALORIES FROM   PRO-37%/CARB-33%/FAT-30%

Ingredients:

1 serving (2 scoops) Vanilla Protein Powder
1 c   Nonfat Milk
1 c   Three Berries (frozen berry mix from Costco—raspberries,
           blueberries, marionberries)
6 Raw   Almonds
1 t   Olive Oil
1 T   Flaxseed Meal

Instructions:

Blend with about six ice cubes, a few at a time, in blender for desired consistency.

Get Your Greens On Smoothie

Makes 1 Serving

NUTRITION PROFILE   CAL-224/PRO-25/CARB-20/FAT-5/SAT-0/
                           CHO-12/SOD-105/FIB-6
PERCENT CALORIES FROM   PRO-43%/CARB-35%/FAT-22%

Ingredients:

½ c	Pomegranate Juice
1/3 c	Raspberries
1/3 c	Strawberries
1/3 c	Blueberries
1 t	Lemon Juice
1 c	Baby Spinach
1 Scoop	Vanilla Protein Powder
Ice Cubes	

Instructions:

Blend with about six ice cubes, a few at a time, in blender for desired consistency.

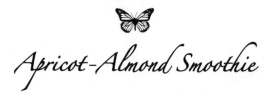

Apricot-Almond Smoothie

Makes 2 Servings

NUTRITION PROFILE   CAL-206/PRO-20/CARB-28/FAT-6/SAT-0/
CHO-8/SOD-160/FIB-3
PERCENT CALORIES FROM   PRO-31%/CARB-46%/FAT-23%

Ingredients:

4	Apricots, pitted
½ c	Carrot Juice
1/2 c	Non Fat Plain Yogurt
1 Scoop	(1/2 serving) Vanilla Protein Powder
1 T	Honey or Agave Nectar
8	Raw Almonds

Instructions:

Blend with about six ice cubes, a few at a time, in blender for desired consistency.

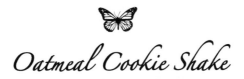

Oatmeal Cookie Shake

Makes 1 Serving

The texture of this shake is a bit chunky, and if you partially blend it, you tidbits of raisins, nuts and oats will surprise the palette.

NUTRITION PROFILE	CAL-286/PRO-29/CARB-34/FAT-4/SAT-0/
	CHO-13/SOD-61/FIB-2
PERCENT CALORIES FROM	PRO-39%/CARB-47%/FAT-14%

Ingredients:

2 T	Rolled Oats
1 scoop	Vanilla Protein Powder
2 t	Raisins
2 t Raw	Walnuts (or Almonds)
½ c	Nonfat Milk or Vanilla Rice Dream
½ t	Cinnamon
2 t	Honey or Agave Nectar
Ice Cubes	

Instructions:

Blend with about six ice cubes, a few at a time, in blender for desired consistency. Add a small amount of water if you prefer a more fluid texture.

Satisfying Sides
(that won't give you big thighs!)

Patti's Quinoa Salad

Makes 8 Servings

NUTRITION PROFILE   CAL-157/PRO-6/CARB-27/FAT-3/SAT-0/
                           CHO-0/SOD-13/FIB-5
PERCENT CALORIES FROM   PRO-15%/CARB-67%/FAT-18%

Ingredients:

2 c   Quinoa (cook per package instructions)
2 large   Red Bell Peppers
2 large   Cucumbers, peeled
4   Green Onions, sliced
2 cups   Baby Carrots
2   Lemons, juiced
1 t   Olive Oil
Salt and Pepper to taste

Instructions:

Prepare the Quinoa as directed on package and allow to cool.
Dice vegetables and add to quinoa. Then add the olive oil, lemon juice, and salt and pepper to taste.

Serving suggestion: Although Quinoa is naturally protein rich balance individual requirements by serving with chicken kabobs, tuna patties or other lean protein source.

🦋

Southern Greens Gone Clean

Makes 12 Servings

Using a variety of textures and flavors, this dish makes these hearty greens easy on the palette. The greens are available in your standard grocery stores, usually bagged. Use the three varieties listed below, or just your favorites. Curly Mustard has a pungent peppery-mustard flavor, while Collard has a broccoli-cabbage like flavor. Country Greens is a mix of southern greens including collard, mustard and turnip. You will need one and one-half bags total for the recipe.

NUTRITION PROFILE	CAL-78/PRO-3/CARB-13/FAT-2/SAT-0/
	CHO-1/SOD-103/FIB-3
PERCENT CALORIES FROM	PRO-13%/CARB-62%/FAT-25%

Ingredients:

1	Yellow Onions, Chopped
2	Garlic Cloves
1/2 c	Sundried Figs, Chopped
1 c	Sundried Tomatoes (or 2 T Tomato Paste to substitute)
1 c	Chicken Stock
1 T	Blackstrap Molasses
1 T	Agave Nectar or Honey
1 T	Pomegranate Balsamic Vinegar
	(or any red wine vinegar to substitute)
1 t	Olive Oil
1 t	Crushed Red Peppers
½ t	Nature Seasoning (blend of herbs and spices or substitute with salt)

1 ½   Bag Collard Greens, Curly Mustard or Country Mix, or
any combination of the three

½ c   Pomegranate Aerials (seeds)

¼ c   Roasted Slivered Almonds, unsalted

In large wok or skillet, add olive oil and sauté onions until translucent, then add garlic.

Stir in ½ bag of greens and 1 cup chicken stock to reduce greens. Add the remaining greens as you have space in the skillet. Continue with the figs, sundried tomatoes, molasses, vinegar, Nature Seasoning and peppers and cook through. Garnish with slivered almonds and pomegranate seeds.

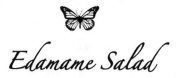

Edamame Salad

Makes 8 Servings

NUTRITION PROFILE   CAL-163/PRO-11/CARB-19/FAT-5/SAT-1/
CHO-0/SOD-80/FIB-5

PERCENT CALORIES FROM   PRO-27%/CARB-45%/FAT-28%

Ingredients:

1 Package	Frozen Edamame (shelled soy beans), thawed
½	Red Onion, Finely Chopped
1 Package	Frozen Corn
¼ c	Fresh Cilantro, Chopped
2	Grated Carrots
2 t	Serrano Pepper, finely chopped

Dressing:

3 t	Grated Fresh Ginger or 2 t Powdered Ginger
2 T	Lemon Juice
1 T	Lemon Zest
¼ t	Soy Sauce (low sodium)
¼ t	Ground Cayenne

Instructions:

Thaw soy beans in strainer under cold running water. Combine all main ingredients. In separate bowl, mix dressing ingredients. Combine. Garnish with Cilantro.

Time Saving Tip: Replace dressing ingredients with Newman's Own Low Fat Ginger Soy Dressing It's healthy, easy and delicious!

Mango, Corn and Black Bean Salad

Makes 4 servings

NUTRITION PROFILE   CAL-145/PRO-4/CARB-25/FAT-4/SAT-1/
                       CHO-0/SOD-319/FIB-5

PERCENT CALORIES FROM PRO-11%/CARB-64%/FAT-25%

Ingredients:

Dressing

1 T	Olive Oil
½ t	Salt
½ t	Garlic Powder
2 t	Dijon Mustard
½ t	Black Pepper
1 T	Lime Juice
2 T	Fresh Cilantro, chopped fine

Salad

6 c.	Mixed Salad Greens
½ c	Black Beans, such as Bearitos Fat Free Black Beans
1 c	Corn Kernels, either fresh or frozen (cooked, thawed)
1	Mango, peeled and cubed

Instructions:

Combine first seven ingredients and mix well. Refrigerate. Place prepared salad greens, black beans, corn kernels, and mango in salad bowl. Pour dressing over salad and serve.

Time Saving Tip: In place of dressing, use Newman's Light Ginger Sesame Dressing.

NewsBite: Salad bars giving you saddle bags?

Avoid the prepared salads with heavy dressings and opt instead for building your own using a base of fresh spinach, romaine lettuce and colorful veggies. And bring your own dressing. Who knows what evil lurks in that salad dressing bin with the greasy ladle? There are several dressing sprits bottles on the market. Carrying a whopping 1 calorie per sprits, you can afford to eat more than iceberg lettuce. This can make the difference between a high calorie and clean eating meal. And it fits conveniently in most small purses.

Healthy Hummus with Veggie Spears

Makes 6 Servings

NUTRITION PROFILE   CAL-135/PRO-6/CARB-25/FAT-2/SAT-0/
CHO-0/SOD-438/FIB-6

PERCENT CALORIES FROM   PRO-13%/CARB-71%/FAT-16%

Ingredients:

1 can	Garbanzo Beans, reserve water from can for desired consistency
¼ c	Nonfat Greek Yogurt (or substitute plain, nonfat yogurt, any variety)
1 t	Pepper
1 t	Garlic Powder
1 t	Ground Cumin
1 t	Cayenne Pepper
½ t	Salt
1 t	Olive Oil
2	Cucumbers, unpeeled
3	Red Bell Pepper
4	Carrots

Instructions:

Blend in food processor. Add reserved liquid from beans for desired consistency. Serve with sliced cucumber, red bell pepper and carrot spears.

Apple-Carrot Salad with Walnuts

Makes 4 Servings

This dish is crunchy and refreshing. The sweet bits of cranberries compliment the slightly tart yogurt. Grated carrots can be purchased at the store or you can grate them yourself and burn a few extra calories while you're at it. If you buy them purchased, be sure to chop them slightly as their length makes for an unmanageable fork-full!

NUTRITION PROFILE	CAL-147/PRO-7/CARB-29/FAT-2/SAT-0/
	CHO-2/SOD-99/FIB-3
PERCENT CALORIES FROM	PRO-17%/CARB-73%/FAT-10%

Ingredients:

2 c	Carrots, Grated
2	Apples, Chopped with Skin
1 c	Nonfat Plain Yogurt
¼ c	Dried Cranberries
1 T	Chopped Walnuts

Instructions: Combine in small bowl and stir. Use this as a crunchy Baja-style taco topper! Add a little grilled chicken to a 100% whole wheat tortilla and top with the salad. It's not only fulfilling but d'lish!

Heirloom Tomato, Jicima and Cucumber Salad in Spicy Lime Vinaigrette

NUTRITION PROFILE	CAL-142/PRO-4/CARB-16/FAT-7/SAT-0/ CHO-0/SOD-109/FIB-4
PERCENT CALORIES FROM	PRO-11%/CARB-43%/FAT-46%

Ingredients:

- 3 c   Romaine Lettuce, chopped
- 15   Heirloom Tomatoes (or Cherry)
- 1 c   Jicima, peeled and cubed
- ½ c   English Cucumber, peeled and sliced
- ¼ c   Garbanzo Beans
- 1 T   Fresh Basil, chopped
- 1 T   Lime Juice
- ½ t   Cayenne Pepper
- 1 T   Olive Oil
- 1 T   White Wine Vinegar

Instructions:

For dressing, mix lime juice, cayenne pepper, fresh basil, olive oil and vinegar. Assemble romaine lettuce on plates and garnish with tomatoes, jicima, cucumbers and garbanzo beans. Dress with lime vinaigrette and serve. Serving Suggestion: Top with 3 oz broiled Salmon or Chicken Breast

Van Gough Veggie Salad

Makes 12 servings

NUTRITION PROFILE   CAL-74/PRO-3/CARB-14/FAT-1/SAT-1/
CHO-0/SOD-306/FIB-4

PERCENT CALORIES FROM   PRO-13%/CARB-71%/FAT-16%

When you make your food look like a work of art, such as impressionist artists Van Gough or Monet, with their clearly defined and brilliant brush strokes of vibrant color, you will pack in a greater variety of nutrients. Imagine the orange bell pepper contrasted with the violets in cabbage and the green cucumber peel . . . the more color the greater variety of nutrients and appeal to your palette! This salad keeps well in the refrigerator for several days.

Ingredients:

3 c	Red Cabbage
2	small Zucchini
3 c	Cauliflower
5	Scallions
3	Carrots
2	Orange Bell Peppers
2	Red Bell Peppers
1	Cucumber
1 c	Sweet Peas
Dash Pepper	
6 oz.	Leftover Chicken Breast, grilled and cubed
1 c	Newman's Own Low Fat Sesame Ginger Dressing

Instructions:

Chop or grate all ingredients through food processor. Add Newman's
Own Light Sesame Ginger dressing then toss and serve.
Top with grilled chicken breast

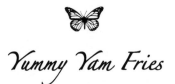

Yummy Yam Fries

Makes 4 Servings

NUTRITION PROFILE   CAL-105/PRO-1/CARB-20/FAT-2/SAT-0/
                          CHO-0/SOD-7/FIB-3
PERCENT CALORIES FROM   PRO-5%/CARB-73%/FAT-22%

Also known as PMS fries . . . naturally sweet, salty, crunchy and spicy, cravings never tasted so good! Nix the drive-through fries, these are good for you!

Ingredients:

2 medium	Sweet Potatoes peeled (Jewel Yams)
1 T	Olive Oil
2	Fresh Garlic Cloves, minced or 1 T Garlic Powder
½ t	Ground Cayenne Red Pepper
1 T	Ground Thyme
Salt	

Instructions:

Pre-heat oven to 350. Peel yams then cut in half crosswise. Cut into 2-3" long by ½" wide fries. Cutting these buggers can be a little tricky. They have a firm consistency and splinter when they are cut. Use a large sharp knife. It may take a time or two to master the technique, but once you get it, it's quite easy. You can also "cube" them if you prefer. Just as tasty but no longer "finger food"!

In a bowl, coat fries with olive oil, then toss with remaining ingredients. Spray baking sheet with nonstick cooking spray. Arrange fries in single layer and bake at 350 for about 30 minutes. Turn fries over and cook another 15-30 minutes until browned.

Time Saving Tip: Too hungry to wait? Microwave the fries for 8 minutes, then coat with spices. Bake for 30 minutes or longer, until crisp.

Quinoa, Brown Rice and Mushroom Medley

Makes 16 Servings (3/4 cup)

NUTRITION PROFILE	CAL-137/PRO-5/CARB-27/FAT-1/SAT-0/
	CHO-1/SOD-122/FIB-4
PERCENT CALORIES FROM	PRO-15%/CARB-79%/FAT-6%

Ingredients:

3 c	Uncooked Trader Joe's Brown Rice Medley (or substitute any whole grain brown rice)
1 c	Uncooked Quinoa
2 c	Organic Chicken Broth or equivalent (TJ) (C)
1 Pkg.	Dried Wild Mushrooms (Porcini, Shiitake, Black & Oyster) or substitute 2 c Fresh Mushrooms chopped, any variety
¼ c	Green Onions, Chopped or 1 T Freeze Dried Shallots
¼ t	Black Pepper
2 c	Water

Instructions:

Finely chop mushrooms. Rinse quinoa then add rice, quinoa and two cups chicken broth to rice cooker. Top off with water to 4 cup fill line. Add mushrooms and green onions. Cover and cook.

Maple-Cinnamon Yams

Makes 10 Servings

NUTRITION PROFILE   CAL-211/PRO-2.5/CARB-49.9/FAT-0/
                                        SAT-0/CHO-1/SOD-477/FIB-7
PERCENT CALORIES FROM   PRO-5%/CARB-94%/FAT-1%

Ingredients:

4	Large Yams, peeled and cubed
1/8 c	Pure Maple Syrup
2 t	Cinnamon
1 T	Vanilla
½ c	Nonfat Milk or Dairy Free Vanilla Rice Dream
1 t	Salt

Instructions:

Peel and cube yams and microwave them with a little water, in a covered dish, until cooked through, about 25 minutes. Drain any water and mash. Add Vanilla Rice Dream for desired moistness and consistency. Add syrup, cinnamon and salt. (Mix everything by hand with a potato masher; if you use beaters the smoother texture isn't as good).

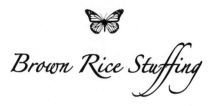

Brown Rice Stuffing

Makes 12 Servings

NUTRITION PROFILE   CAL-181/PRO-5/CARB-35/FAT-3/SAT-0/
                          CHO-1/SOD-164/FIB-2
PERCENT CALORIES FROM   PRO-10%/CARB-74%/FAT-16%

Ingredients:

2 c	Trader Joe's Brown Rice Medley (TJ)
	(A blend of long-grain brown rice, black barley and daikon radish seeds) or equivalent
¾ c	Quinoa (G) (WF)
1	Yellow Onion
2	Cloves Garlic
1 T	Olive Oil
½ c	Dried Cranberries
1 T	Walnuts, chopped
1 T	Grated Orange Peel
3 ½ c	Swanson Low Sodium Chicken Broth or TJ's Organic

Instructions:

In saucepan, stir fry onion and garlic. Add TJ's Brown Rice and Quinoa and stir until mixed well. Add broth and simmer for 30 minutes. Add dried cranberries, orange peel and walnuts and allow to simmer until cooked through. Serving Suggestion: Pair with a lean protein and vegetable for a balanced meal

Creamy Cauliflower Soup

Makes 6 Servings

NUTRITION PROFILE   CAL-64/PRO-6/CARB-7/FAT-2/SAT-0/
CHO-2/SOD-240/FIB-22

PERCENT CALORIES FROM   PRO-30/CARB-48%/FAT-22%

Ingredients:

1	Head Cauliflower
1	Yellow Onion, cut into wedges
2 c	Trader Joe's Free Range Chicken Broth or Fat Free Chicken Broth
1 c	Nonfat Milk
2	Stalks Celery
2 T	Parmesan Cheese, finely grated
5	Garlic Cloves, peeled, whole
1 t	Salt
1 t	White Pepper (or black as substitute)
1 T	Herbes de Province (dried herb blend found at most grocery stores)
1 t	Olive Oil

Chives, Chopped

Optional: You can use almost any squash type vegetable to this dish, such as yellow crookneck or zucchini. Experiment!

Instructions:

Remove inner core and leaves from cauliflower and break into florets. In a medium pot, add 3 ½ cups of water and bring to boil. Steam cauliflower, chopped celery, garlic cloves and onion until tender.

Reserve ½ cup cooking water. In a blender, and working in two batches, add half the cauliflower, onion and garlic mixture, ½ cup milk and 1 cup chicken broth and blend until smooth. In last blender batch, add remaining nonfat milk, chicken broth, parmesan cheese olive oil, and salt and pepper. Blend until smooth. Add reserved ½ cup of cooking water for desired consistency if needed. Pour all back into original pot and stir to blend, while reheating. Garnish with fresh chives.

Optional Cooking Tool: Immersion blenders allow you to effortless cream your soups right in the pot you are cooking. Put it on your Christmas gift list!

Toni's Roasted Bell Pepper Tomato Soup

Makes 6, 2 cup servings

NUTRITION PROFILE   CAL-145/PRO-10/CARB-21/FAT-3/SAT-1/
CHO-5/SOD-388/FIB-4

PERCENT CALORIES FROM   PRO-25/CARB-55%/FAT-20%

Ingredients:

1	Medium Yellow Onion, chopped
½ c	Chopped Carrots
2	Stalks Celery, chopped
2 t	Olive Oil
3 ½ lbs	(about 13) Ripe Tomatoes (or substitute 28 oz. Can Whole Tomatoes, un-drained)
14 oz	Organic Chicken Broth or Chicken Stock (low sodium)
1 t	Salt
½ t	Ground Pepper
7	Cloves Garlic, chopped
½ c	Nonfat Milk
2 T	Romano or Parmesan Cheese, grated
8 oz Jar	Roasted Bell Peppers, drained (packed in water, not oil)
1 cup	Nonfat Cottage Cheese
Salt to taste	

Instructions:

If using fresh tomatoes, blanch in boiling water for 30 seconds until skin splits. Remove skins, quarter and remove core. In saucepan, cook onion, carrots, celery and garlic in the olive oil. Add fresh or canned tomatoes and broth. Cook on medium heat for 20 minutes. Add nonfat milk. Add pepper, grated cheese, cottage cheese and drained roasted red peppers. Use immersion blender (or regular blender in small batches) until smooth.

Green Beans with Apricots and Almonds

Makes 4 Servings

NUTRITION PROFILE	CAL-84/PRO-2/CARB-12/FAT-3/SAT-0/
	CHO-5/SOD-712/FIB-4
PERCENT CALORIES FROM	PRO-10/CARB-54%/FAT-36%

This is a light and healthy side dish with delicate flavors.

Ingredients:

1 pound	Green Beans, trimmed and sliced in 1" diagonal strips
2	Cloves Fresh Garlic, minced or 2 t Garlic Powder
3T	Sliced Almonds
1 t	Olive Oil
4	Fresh Apricots stem and pit removed or 4 T
	Dried Apricots, chopped
1 t	Salt
½ t	Pepper

Preparation:

First blanch the beans, cook them in a pot of boiling, salted water until a dente, about 5 minutes. Do not cover the pot. Drain well, and then toss while warm in the olive oil, garlic, salt and pepper.

Spread sliced almonds in single layer on sheet and toast in oven on 350 until lightly toasted.

Cut fresh apricots in half and remove the pit. Slice into strips and set aside.

Assemble the warm beans, apricot cubes, toasted almonds and salt and pepper, and then toss gently in a bowl. Serve immediately.

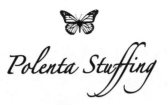

Polenta Stuffing

Makes 12 Servings

NUTRITION PROFILE   CAL-226/PRO-6/CARB-40/FAT-5/SAT-0/
CHO-30/SOD-198/FIB-3

PERCENT CALORIES FROM   PRO-10/CARB-71%/FAT-19%

For holidays, or anytime, this is a truly satisfying dish. If you make the corn bread a day or ahead, it actually works well because it displaces the traditional crunchy crouton. Get a jump on your entertaining by making the corn bread and freezing it for later use! The nutritional profile contains the macronutrients for the corn bread and stuffing mixture combined.

For the Polenta Corn Bread

3	Egg Whites
1 1/3 c	Nonfat Milk or Rice Dream
2 c	Golden Pheasant Polenta
1 c	Fresh or Frozen Corn Kernels (defrosted)
1 T	Canola Oil
1½ c	Oat Flour or Bob's GF Flour (WF) (B)
1 T	Baking Powder
½ t	Salt
2 T	Agave Nectar

Mix flours, baking powder and salt in bowl. Add egg whites, milk, canola oil and agave nectar. Mix until blended. Add polenta (corn meal) and mix thoroughly. Bake at 325 until cooked about 20-30 minutes. Test with toothpick and allow to cool.

Stuffing

1/3 c	Walnuts
2 Stalks	Celery, chopped
1	Yellow Onion
1	Grated Orange Rind
1/3 c	Triple Sec
1 c	Dried Cranberries
2 T	chopped Fresh Parsley
2 t	Chopped Fresh Thyme
2 c	Trader Joe's Organic Chicken Broth
1 t	Salt

Instructions:

Once corn bread is cooled, break into small chunks. Spray frying pan with nonstick cooking spray, and fry yellow onion and celery. Place in casserole dish and add remaining dry ingredients, and gently fold in corn bread chunks. Sprinkle chicken broth, then triple sec over mixture and bake at 350 for 20 minutes in covered dish.

Fulfilling Feasts

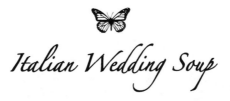

Italian Wedding Soup

Makes 8 Servings

NUTRITION PROFILE   CAL-255/PRO-17/CARB-38/FAT-5/SAT-0/
                         CHO-30/SOD-219/FIB-8
PERCENT CALORIES FROM   PRO-25/CARB-58%/FAT-17%

Meatball Ingredients:

1 Pkg (11 oz)	Jenny-O Lean Ground Turkey or equivalent
½ c	Oat Bran
2 T	Paresano-Reggiano Cheese, finely grated
2 t	Garlic Powder, or 5 Cloves
2 t	Dried Basil
1 t	Ground Cloves
¼ c	Fresh Parsley, chopped
2	Egg Whites
1 t	Salt
½ t	Black Ground Pepper

Soup Ingredients:

1 49.5oz Can	Swanson's 99% Fat Free Chicken Broth
3 c	Fresh Spinach
8 oz.	Rice Select Orzo Whole Wheat Pasta
1 T	Parmesan Cheese

Instructions:

Combine all meatball ingredients and roll into 1" diameter balls. In non-stick pan, spray Pam or equivalent. Cook meatballs until browned, not cooked through.

In large pot, add chicken broth and meatballs, then cook on medium heat for 10 minutes. Add orzo and spinach, cook another 10 minutes until pasta is cooked a dente, stirring occasionally. Sprinkle with the remaining 1 tablespoon parmesan cheese and serve. Molto bene!

Turkey Loaf

Makes 8 Servings

NUTRITION PROFILE   CAL-182/PRO-19/CARB-12/FAT-6/SAT-2/
                        CHO-55/SOD-211/FIB-2
PERCENT CALORIES FROM   PRO-42/CARB-26%/FAT-32%

Ingredients:

1 lb	Lean Ground Turkey
½ c	Oat Bran or Rolled Oats
1	Yellow Onion, chopped
½ c	Celery, chopped
2 T	Sundried Tomatoes, chopped
1 t	Garlic Powder
1 T	Basil fresh, or 2 t dried
1 T	Ground Cumin
1 t	Crushed Red Pepper
1/3 c	Mint Leaves, finely chopped
1 t	Pepper
1 T	Parmesan Cheese
2 Large	Egg Whites
2	Scallions, finely chopped
1 c	Mushrooms, sliced
2 T	Organic Ketchup

Instructions:

In food processor, pulse ground turkey, rolled oats, yellow onion, celery, mushrooms and seasonings, including mint. In bowl add egg, scallions, parmesan cheese, and sundried tomatoes. Spray a bread loaf pan with nonstick cooking spray and bake at 350 for 40-45 minutes. Remove and top with ¼ cup organic ketchup and bake for another 5-7 minutes. Take out and let cool before serving.

Barbequed Turkey Breast in Yogurt-Jalapeno Marinade

Makes 12 Servings (approx 4 oz each)

NUTRITION PROFILE CAL-139/PRO-29/CARB-2/FAT-1/SAT-0/
         CHO-71/SOD-75/FIB-0

PERCENT CALORIES FROM PRO-89/CARB-6%/FAT-5%

Ingredients:

3 lbs Turkey Breast, boned and halved, thawed partially
1 c Greek Yogurt or Plain Nonfat Yogurt
1 T Jalapeno pepper, Minced and seeded
1 t Cumin
1/4 t Cayenne Pepper
1/8 t Nutmeg
1/8 t Garlic Powder

Instructions:

Remove skin and all fat from turkey breast. Butterfly the breast by using a sharp knife; start in the center of the long side and cut in half to within about ½" of other long side. Open meat flat and set on platter.

Mix together yogurt, and all spices in a small bowl. Rub mixture over turkey, cover, and chill overnight or at least for a couple of hours to marinate. Grill meat 4 inches from heat source until cooked through, about 10 minutes per side. Check by piercing meat; juice should be clear and no longer pink. Let stand for 5 minutes, then cut diagonally into slices. Serving Suggestion: Serve with Yummy Yam Fries and Green Beans with Apricots for a perfectly balanced meal!

Honey-Almond Salmon over Mixed Greens

Makes 4 Servings

NUTRITION PROFILE   CAL-286/PRO-29/CARB-14/FAT-12/SAT-2/
                                CHO-60/SOD-122/FIB-3

PERCENT CALORIES FROM   PRO-41%/CARB-20%/FAT-39%

Ingredients:

2 T	Almond Meal (WF) (TJS)
1 T	Raw Almonds
1 T	Honey or Agave Nectar
1 T	Red Pepper Flakes
1 T	Kirkland Sweet Mesquite Seasoning (C)
2 6 oz.	Wild Salmon Fillets (C) (G) (WF) (TJS)
1 T	Fresh Basil, Chopped or ½ t dried basil
Dash Salt (to taste)	
4 c	Mixed Baby Greens
1 c	Heirloom Tomatoes (TJS)
	Or Cherry Tomatoes (G)
1 c	Cucumbers, Sliced (any variety below)
	Persian (TJS)
	English (C)
	Regular (G)
1 t	Olive Oil
2 t	Balsamic Vinegar

Instructions:

Thaw salmon and pat dry. Brush honey on top of each filet. Mix red pepper flakes, mesquite seasoning and almond meal in a bowl. Sprinkle with red pepper flakes, then coat with almond meal and top with coarsely chopped almonds. Sprinkle with fresh or dried Basil. Broil or bake for about 15 minutes. Finished when salmon flakes in center.

Assemble baby greens on each plate. Drizzle with the olive oil and vinegar. Cut tomatoes in half and arrange with cucumbers. Add cooked salmon on top and garnish with basil leaves and a few remaining tomatoes.

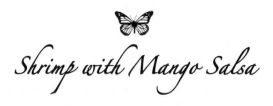

Shrimp with Mango Salsa

Makes 4 Servings

NUTRITION PROFILE   CAL-272/PRO-36/CARB-224/FAT-4/SAT-1/
CHO-259/SOD-542/FIB-2
PERCENT CALORIES FROM   PRO-52%/CARB-33%/FAT-15%

Ingredients:

Salsa:
2 large	Ripe Mangoes, peeled, pitted, and diced
¼ c	Minced Red Onion
¼ c	Chopped Cilantro Leaves
3 T	Fresh Lime Juice
1 t	Minced Fresh Ginger
¼ t	Freshly Ground Black Pepper

Shrimp:
1 ½	Pounds Large Shrimp, peeled and deveined (C)
2 T	Reduced-Sodium Soy Sauce
2 T	Fresh Orange Juice
½ T	Olive Oil

Instructions:

To make salsa: Combine all ingredients in a bowl. Set aside. To make shrimp: Rinse and drain shrimp; pat dry with paper towels. In a bowl, combine shrimp, soy sauce, and orange juice. Let stand 10 minutes. Stir fry using only enough olive oil to lightly coat the pan. Serving Suggestion: Serve with mango salsa and brown rice medley.

Ahi Hoke Poke (pronounced Hokie Pokie)

Makes 4 Servings

NUTRITION PROFILE   CAL-224/PRO-31/CARB-16/FAT-4/SAT-1/
                           CHO-51/SOD-896/FIB-3

PERCENT CALORIES FROM   PRO-55%/CARB-29%/FAT-16%

Ingredients:

2	English Cucumbers, Peeled, Halved, and Finely Sliced
1/3 C	Seasoned Rice Vinegar
½ C	Low Salt Soy Sauce
½ C	Chopped Green Onions
1 T	Sesame Oil
1 T	Black (preferably) or White Toasted Sesame Seeds
1 T	Chili Sauce
1/2 Can	(8 Oz) Water Chestnuts, Chopped
1 Lb	FRESH Sushi Grade Ahi Tuna Cut into ¾" Cubes
1	Whole Wheat Pita Chips for Garnish

Instructions:

Finely slice cucumbers and remove seeds if desired. Marinate in refrigerator for one hour in seasoned rice vinegar. Combine sesame oil, chili sauce and soy sauce. Set aside. Freeze Ahi Tuna steak for about 10 minutes, just until firm to make cutting easier. Cut into ¾" cubes and combine marinate in soy sauce, sesame oil and chili sauce for one hour. Fold in chopped water chestnuts. Cut whole wheat pita into eight equal triangles and toast. Assemble by placing sliced cucumbers in a martini glass. Top with Ahi then sprinkle with green onions and sesame seeds. Garnish with three pita chips. Serve immediately.

How to select fresh tuna: Always make sure it is sushi grade. It may be purchased as a steak either fresh or frozen. I enjoy purchasing it from our local farmers market. Avoid any with dry or brown spots (other than the natural darker brown area). There should be no rainbow sheen on the fish and should smell ocean-fresh. If you have the option, skip the thawed frozen filets and buy the tuna filet frozen. This way, you know it will be the freshest possible since you control when to thaw it. Just be sure to store it in the coldest part of your freezer until you're ready to thaw. Keep the tuna refrigerated until you're ready to use it. It's best to use fresh tuna the day of purchase. If you need to store it, pat it dry, wrap securely in plastic wrap or foil and store in the coldest part of your refrigerator (optimum temperature of 31 degrees F.). If your refrigerator is not that cold, place the wrapped fish on a bed of ice or in a baggie filled with ice. Use within 24 hours.

Chicken Satay with Peanut Sauce

Makes 6 servings (two skewers per serving)

NUTRITION PROFILE	CAL-160/PRO-26/CARB-6/FAT-4/SAT-1/
	CHO-65/SOD-879/FIB-0
PERCENT CALORIES FROM	PRO-62/CARB-14/FAT-24%

Ingredients:

Marinade:

6	Boneless Chicken Breasts, cubed and uncooked
2 T	Curry Powder
1 T	Honey or Agave Nectar
1 T	Olive Oil
1/4 c	Low Salt Soy Sauce
4	Garlic Cloves, finely chopped

Peanut Sauce

3/4 c	Organic Chicken Broth, Fat Free, Reduced Sodium
1 1/3 c	PB2 or Substitute
2	Cloves Garlic Finely Chopped or 1 T Powdered Garlic
1 ½ T	Lemon Juice
½ t	Paprika (mild) or Cayenne (spicy hot)
6-8	Bamboo Skewers, soaked in water for 30 minutes

Marinate for two hours. Then thread on bamboo skewers and cook in oven, broil, or over charcoal. On stovetop add chicken broth, PB2 and chopped garlic. Cook for a few minutes until it thickens. Remove from heat and add remaining ingredients. Enjoy this sinless indulgence! Serving Suggestion: Serve with Brown Rice Stuffing and Creamy Cauliflower Soup!

Stuffed Mexican Zucchini

Makes 6 Servings

NUTRITION PROFILE   CAL-247/PRO-22/CARB-25/FAT-7/SAT-2/
                                    CHO-55/SOD-794/FIB-5
PERCENT CALORIES FROM   PRO-35/CARB-40%/FAT-25%

What a great way to get your family to eat their vegetables without it being obvious! Mexican zucchini are fun in their small, pumpkin-shapes. If these are not available, any variety of zucchini will work just fine. Because each serving is completely balanced with lean protein, complex carbohydrates and healthy fat they can be served as a single entrée. You may have extra "stuffing" remaining. If so, bake in a separate casserole dish along with the zucchini. This too, is included in the nutrient profile so you may add one sixth to your plate.

Ingredients:

6 Round	Mexican or 3 regular Zucchini Squash
½ c	Chopped Onion
3	Cloves Garlic
1 lb.	Lean Ground Turkey meat
½ c	Grated carrots
2 c	cooked Quinoa/Brown Rice
3	Egg Whites
½ c	CLASSICO di Napoli Tomato & Basil Pasta Sauce (or equivalent)
Cayenne Pepper	
½ t	Salt
1 T	Grated Parmesan Cheese

Instructions:

For the round variety, cut off the top with stem and set aside. For the oblong zucchini, cut it in half lengthwise. Using a spoon, scoop out the flesh of the vegetable, leaving about ¼" of the shell and set both aside. In a skillet, cook chopped onion and garlic until caramelized. Add brown ground turkey meat chopped onion, garlic and salt and cook through. Add zucchini flesh previously scooped out and cook into the meat mixture. In a separate bowl, combine leftover brown rice/quinoa mixture, grated carrots, egg whites, salt and pepper. Mix well by hand. Fold the turkey mixture into the rice mixture until combined. Stuff each round or halved zucchini with mixture and use pressure to compact. Top with tomato sauce and sprinkling of parmesan cheese. Bake in 350 degree oven for 45 minutes, or until zucchini can be pierced easily with a fork.

Turkey-Bean Chile with Brown Rice, Pearl Barley and Quinoa

Makes 28 Servings (approx 1 cup)

NUTRITION PROFILE	CAL-174/PRO-13/CARB-25/FAT-3/SAT-1/
	CHO-0/SOD-102/FIB-5
PERCENT CALORIES FROM	PRO-30%/CARB-56%/FAT-14%

This heart-warming and fulfilling dish combines rice and beans and complex flavors, creating a perfect protein as it contains all the essential amino acids. Quinoa is high in protein so for a vegetarian option simply eliminate the ground turkey. I recently brought this dish to my nephew Charles' 27th birthday and because it is so healthy and hearty, was warmly received by all his dirt bike riding buddies.

Rather than add uncooked barley, rice and quinoa to the broth, I prefer to add leftover cooked grains. This helps balance out the amount of liquid so I can decide to make it more of a soup or a chunky stew. The latter is my ultimate favorite.

Ingredients:

4 c	Assorted Dried Beans
	(Such as Bob's Red Mill 13 Bean Soup or Mix Your Own—see below for instructions*)
2 32 oz	Cartons Organic Chicken Broth or Low Sodium Equivalent
1	Chopped Medium Yellow Onion or 5 Green Onions
2 cans	(14.5 oz each) Stewed Tomatoes
2 packages	Ground Lean Turkey

1 c	Yellow Corn
3 T	Chile Powder
1 T	Molasses
8	Cloves Garlic or 1 T Garlic Powder
3 T	Ground Cumin
4 T	Lime Juice
2 T	Sriracha sauce (Asian Hot Chile Sauce)
Salt to Taste	
1 c	Cooked Pearl Barley
1 c	Cooked Brown Rice
1 c	Cooked Quinoa

Instructions:

Setting this up in the morning in a crock pot is a time saving way to prepare this meal. No overnight soaking of the beans required. Simply rinse and drain dried beans. In crock pot, soak beans in chicken broth. In separate pan lightly sprayed with nonfat cooking spray, brown ground turkey, onions and garlic, drain off any oils, and add to bean mixture in crock pot. Add remaining ingredients (except for lime juice) and seasonings to taste. Allow to cook all day on low heat. By dinnertime, beans will be cooked through, even if not soaked overnight. Prior to serving add lime juice.

Time Saving Tip: Canned beans are a great option, especially if you do not have a crock pot. Not only do they retain their fiber content and nutritional benefits, but their anti-cancer flavonoids as well. They are quick and easy in comparison to the raw beans long cooking time.

*Mix Your Own!

Buy one package of each type of your favorite dried beans and lentils. The choices are extensive; choose from Pinto, Black, Brown, Red, Garbanzo, Kidney, Lentils, Black Eyed Peas and others from your local grocery store and combine them in a large bowl. Divide into servings of 16 (4 cups each total) and store in large Ziploc bags in your pantry.

Mark each bag with "1 cup = 4 servings" so you can remember the portion size later. Mixing your own gives you a better variety, and saves the cost of pre-packaged mixed beans. Beans have very similar macronutrient profiles and calories, so you don't need to be concerned about which type are accurate for this recipe, just make sure the portion size is the same.

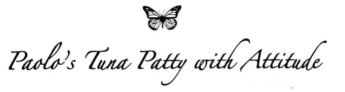

Paolo's Tuna Patty with Attitude

Makes 2 Servings

NUTRITION PROFILE	CAL-237/PRO-34/CARB-11/FAT-5/SAT-1/
	CHO-73/SOD-621/FIB-1
PERCENT CALORIES FROM	PRO-59/CARB-20%/FAT-21%

Ingredients:

6 oz	Raw Ahi Tuna, finely chopped or 1 can (7oz) White Albacore Tuna in water
2 oz.	Wild Smoked Sockeye Salmon, chopped
¼ c	Oats, uncooked, not quick cooking
2	Egg Whites
¼ c	Fresh Italian Parsley or 1 t Dried
½ t	Cumin
2	Green Onions, chopped
½	Serrano Pepper, seeded and chopped
2	Cloves Garlic, chopped

To Garnish:

1 T	Fresh Chives or Italian Parsley
2 T	Nonfat Fage Greek Yogurt (TJ) (WF) (G) or Nonfat Plain Yogurt

Instructions:

Finely chop fresh tuna, or drain canned tuna. In bowl, combine all ingredients except garnishes. Form into two patties by compressing the tuna mixture between the palms of your hands and carefully setting in the pan so they don't fall apart. (Once they begin to cook, they become firm.)

Coat non-stick pan with Pam or equivalent cooking spray. Fry patties on one side on low heat for several minutes until browned. Remove patties from pan and apply nonstick cooking spray before flipping patties to avoid sticking. Top with 1 T each nonfat plain yogurt and sprinkle with chives or parsley. Serving Suggestion: Serve with Heirloom or Cherry Tomatoes. Mangare!

Wendy's Green Chile Chicken Enchiladas

Makes 8 Servings

NUTRITION PROFILE	CAL-262/PRO-21/CARB-43/FAT-5/SAT-1/
	CHO-29/SOD-1016/FIB-12
PERCENT CALORIES FROM	PRO-28/CARB-56%/FAT-16%

One of my dear clients took the initiative to take a clean approach to this traditionally heavy dish. With a few embellishments, such as topping it with nonfat yogurt (which tastes quite similar to sour cream) and adding just a sprinkling of a low fat Mexican cheese for aroma—adding only 10 calories per serving—this has become one our family favorites, thanks to Wendy!

Ingredients:

8	La Tortilla Factory Smart & Delicious 100% Whole Wheat Tortillas
2	Boneless, Skinless Chicken Breasts or Shredded Rotisserie Chicken (breast only, no skin)
1 15 oz can	Low Sodium Black Beans
2 c	Fresh Baby Spinach
1 4 oz can	Fire Roasted Whole Green Chiles (mild)
1 2.25 oz can	Sliced Black Olives (retain a few to top)
1 19 oz can	El Paso Enchilada Sauce (mild)
2 T	Sargento Reduced Fat 4 Cheese Mexican, shredded
½ c	Nonfat Plain Yogurt

Instructions:

Boil chicken breasts until cooked through and shred with fork. Mix together shredded chicken, green chiles, black olives, black beans and one half the enchilada sauce in a medium bowl. Spoon mixture along center of each tortilla and add a few spinach leaves. Roll and place seam-side down in baking dish prepared with nonstick cooking spray. Top with remaining enchilada sauce, a sprinkling of cheese and a few sliced olives. Bake at 350°F for 20 minutes. Garnish with dollop of plain yogurt (one tablespoon per serving)

Stuffed Chicken Breasts with Spinach over Quinoa

Makes 4 Servings

NUTRITION PROFILE	CAL-334/PRO-35/CARB-31/FAT-7/SAT-0/
	CHO-78/SOD-374/FIB-4
PERCENT CALORIES FROM	PRO-42/CARB-38%/FAT-20%

Ingredients:

4	Chicken Breasts, Skinless and Boneless
2 cups	Fresh Spinach Leaves or 1 Pkg. Frozen Spinach, Thawed
½ c	Mushrooms, Chopped
1 T	Parmesan Cheese, Grated
¼ t	Cayenne Pepper
2	Egg Whites
¼ c	Skim Ricotta Cheese
4 Servings	Quinoa (cook per package directions)
99%	Fat Free Chicken Broth, Low Sodium
2 T	Healthy Hummus

Instructions:

Cut pocket in chicken breast, being sure not to cut all the way through the other side. In separate bowl, mix parmesan, ricotta, egg whites and cayenne until thoroughly combined.

Fold in chopped spinach and mushrooms with a dash of salt. Stuff each chicken breast with ¼ of the mixture. Close with a toothpick. Bake at 350 degrees for 40 minutes or electric grill until cooked through. Serve over Quinoa cooked according to package directions, however modify by using 50% low sodium chicken broth and 50%water. Top with about 2 teaspoons of hummus on each chicken breast.

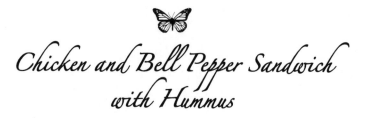

Chicken and Bell Pepper Sandwich with Hummus

Makes 1 serving

NUTRITION PROFILE   CAL-351/PRO-36/CARB-40/FAT-6/SAT-1/
                                      CHO-72/SOD-63/FIB-7

PERCENT CALORIES FROM   PRO-39/CARB-44%/FAT-17%

Ingredients:

Grilled Chicken Breast (3 oz)
3   Roasted Red or Yellow Pepper Quarters
               (Roland or Equivalent) and in a jar not in oil
1 T   Healthy Hummus*
2 Slices   100%Whole Wheat or Ezekiel Bread

*Finding a healthy hummus is key! Many brands are loaded with Tahiti, or sesame oil, which increases the fat and calories substantially. As a guideline, do not exceed 50 calories per serving (2 Tablespoons) and 3 grams of fat maximum. When purchasing from stores, look for 35 calories and 2 grams unsaturated fat per two tablespoons. Better yet, make your own, check out our Healthy Hummus recipe.

Instructions:

Halve the chicken breast lengthwise, to butterfly. When the breasts are half as thick, they cook very quickly. Cook both halves reserving one for another meal.

Time Saving Tip: It's easy to prepare chicken breasts quickly if you have a small electric grill. My preference is the George Foreman Grill, which comes in several sizes. What works best for me is the personal size grill, it's easy to grab out of the cupboard and easy to clean too. It grills chicken, fish, turkey burgers, or veggies in minutes.

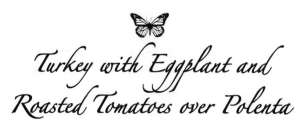

Turkey with Eggplant and Roasted Tomatoes over Polenta

Makes 6 Servings

NUTRITION PROFILE   CAL-165/PRO-17/CARB-20/FAT-2/SAT-0/
                                       CHO-5/SOD-358/FIB-23

PERCENT CALORIES FROM   PRO-39/CARB-47%/FAT-14%

Ingredients:

1	Eggplant, cubed, not peeled
1 ½ c	Mushrooms, quartered
1 12 oz.	Pkg Extra Lean Ground Turkey
4 Vine	Ripened Tomatoes
2 t	Olive Oil
5	Cloves Fresh Garlic, minced or 1 ½ T Garlic Powder
2 t	Dried Basil
1 T	Freeze Dried Shallot, minced
14.5 oz. Can	S&W Italian Recipe Stewed Tomatoes
1 Can	S&W Tomato Sauce
1 t	Black Pepper
2 t	Thyme
Polenta*	

*Trader Joe's makes a delicious Organic Polenta already made. You can choose to make your own as well, which is simple to do. Blue Pheasant makes a dry polenta; an economical and convenient pantry item!

Instructions:

Spray large skillet with nonstick cooking spray. Fry ground turkey and drain oils. Set aside. Using scant amount of olive oil in bottom of pan—just to moisten—fry chopped onions and garlic. Add eggplant and brown. Remove ingredients then core and cut tomatoes in half and place face down in pan, allowing to simmer about 5 minutes until gently roasted. Add can stewed tomatoes and remaining ingredients. Continue to simmer about 10 minutes. Serve over Polenta.

Parmesan Turkey Meatballs with Spaghetti

Makes 6 servings

NUTRITION PROFILE   CAL-303/PRO-25/CARB-42/FAT-3/SAT-1/
CHO-24/SOD-274/FIB-6

PERCENT CALORIES FROM   PRO-33/CARB-57%/FAT-10%

Meatball Ingredients:

1 Pkg (11 oz)	Lean Ground Turkey
½ c	Oat Bran
2 T	Parmesan Cheese, finely grated
2 t	Garlic Powder, or 5 Cloves
2 t	Dried Basil
1 t	Ground Cloves
1 T	Fresh Parsley
1 oz.	Sun Dried Tomatoes (Not in oil)
2	Egg Whites
1 t	Salt
½ t	Black Ground Pepper
1 32 oz. Jar	CLASSICO DiNapoli Tomato & Basil Pasta Sauce*
12 oz.	Whole Wheat Spaghetti (Garfolo or equivalent)

Instructions:

Mix first 11 ingredients into approximately 1" diameter meatballs. Spray non stick frying pan with Pam or equivalent nonstick cooking spray. Brown meatballs; then add sauce and cover until cooked through, about 15 minutes.

Time Saving Tips: Double the batch of meatballs and freeze them to make your next dinner easy. Instead of making your own pasta sauce, use a low fat, healthy alternative, such as Classico DiNapoli Tomato & Basil Pasta Sauce.

A word about whole wheat pastas: as you know, many brands are not created equal and some have the flavor of and consistency of particle board. Some whole wheat pastas now have added protein too. One brand I particularly like, and priced well is found at Costco called Garfolo Spaghetti. Other delicious brands can be found at Trader Joe's and Whole Foods.

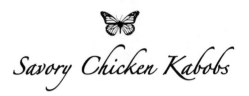

Savory Chicken Kabobs

Makes 6 generous servings

NUTRITION PROFILE	CAL-309/PRO-54/CARB-7/FAT-6/SAT-2/
	CHO-145/SOD-225/FIB-2
PERCENT CALORIES FROM	PRO-72/CARB-9%/FAT-19%

Dry Rub Ingredients:

Seasoning: *(double batch, store half for future use)*

½ t	Ground Cardamom
1 t	Cayenne Pepper
2 t	Ground Coriander
½ t	Ground Cloves
2 T	Ground Ginger
2 T	Ground Cumin

Wet Ingredients:
Single Batch (for use now)

| ½ c | Plain Nonfat Yogurt |
| 2 T | Lemon Juice |

Kabobs:

2	Red Bell Peppers, cut in strips
2	Green Bell Peppers, cut in strips
1 c	Whole Mushrooms
1	Red Onion, cut in strips
6	Boneless Chicken Breasts, each cut into 6 cubes
6	Long Bamboo Skewers

Instructions:

Soak bamboo skewers in water for about 30 minutes to prevent burning on the grill. Mix all ingredients in a glass bowl. If you have the lead time, you can marinate the cubed chicken for 8 hours, otherwise, just lightly coat the chicken and start to skewer! You can grill, roast or stir fry with in a nonstick pan with Pam or equivalent. Serving Suggestion: Serve over brown rice and quinoa.

Time Saving Tip: Make the seasoning in a large batch (dry ingredients only) and keep in your spice cabinet in an airtight container for an effortless and guilt-free seasoning. An advantage of using this spice is you don't have to plan ahead as you don't need to marinate or season in advance, just lightly coat the chicken and start to skewer! These spices seal in the flavor and keep the chicken moist.

Grilled Chicken Breasts with Mango Salsa and Pita Chips

Makes 4 servings

This salsa has a delicious combination of sweet and spicy flavors. It's not only healthy but delicious and worthy to serve at any dinner party. Our kids come back for THIRDS when we have this for dinner!

| NUTRITION PROFILE | CAL-287/PRO-30/CARB-32/FAT-5/SAT-0/CHO-72/SOD-168/FIB-4 |
| PERCENT CALORIES FROM | PRO-41/CARB-43%/FAT-16% |

Ingredients:

2 Mango, Peeled, Remove Seed and Cut Into Cubes
1/4 C Finely Chopped Fresh Cilantro
1/4 C Finely Diced Red Onion
2 T Fresh Lime Juice
1 T Olive Oil
2 t Finely Grated Lime Peel
1 t Finely Chopped Seeded Serrano Chile
Nonstick Vegetable Oil Spray
4 Boneless Chicken Breast Halves Without Skin
2 Whole Wheat Pitas

Instructions:

Combine cubed mango, cilantro, red onion, lime juice, olive oil, grated lime peel, and chopped Serrano Chile in medium bowl. Toss to blend flavors. Season mango salsa to taste with salt and pepper. Spray grill (I use the small double sided George Forman Grill) with nonstick vegetable oil spray; Sprinkle chicken breasts with salt and pepper. Grill chicken breasts until brown and chicken is cooked through, about 5 minutes. Cut whole pita with scissors into eight equal pieces (cut into quarters then cut each quarter in half into triangular chips. Toast until crunchy in toaster oven.

Slice chicken breasts and arrange on plates. Top with mango salsa and cilantro leaves and serve. Serving Suggestion: Use the leftover Mango Salsa over fresh grilled salmon . . . delicious!

CONVERT YOUR FAVORITE RECIPE FROM MEAN TO CLEAN!

Have a delicious recipe that you don't want to abandon but it's not too kind to your thighs? All recipes can be modified by either swapping out the salt, sugar and fat in ingredients to healthier alternatives, switching from overly processed foods to whole grain, and by reducing the amount that is used and using an alternative cooking method such as baking, broiling, and grilling instead of frying or sautéing.

GENERAL MEAN TO BITE ME! CLEAN TIPS:

1. Use a low fat substitute whenever possible for cheeses
2. Reduce the amount of cheese by at least three quarters
3. Use nonfat milk instead of whole
4. Never freely "drizzle" or pour oil on anything. Always measure so you know how much you are eating. For sautéing, moisten a paper towel with a little oil and rub the bottom of the skillet until lightly coated or use nonstick olive or canola oil cooking spray. When a recipe calls for butter, the actual amount needed is about ¼ of what is typically called for.
5. Always switch to whole grains for all pasta, rice and grains
6. Add more vegetables, fresh or frozen spinach is a natural here
7. Reduce the amount of meat. This recipe has enough protein per serving without the full amount.
8. Use as many fresh herbs and spices in all your recipes. They add valuable phytochemicals and health benefits, with next to zero calories.

This original chef's recipe for Turkey Lasagna looks delicious, but high in fat. In fact 43% of the calories are from fat alone. One serving provides 29 grams, which is more than the maximum recommended amount of fat for the entire day!

With the modifications, it provides the perfect balance of protein, carbohydrates and fat, reducing the fat percentage from 41% to 22%.

Aside from the overload of cheese and use of turkey sausage, it includes a savory blend of herbs and spices. It's always rewarding to make your own sauce, but not everyone has that luxury. For a time saving tip, skip the home made sauce and use an organic, low sodium sauce that has all natural ingredients from Trader Joe's or Whole Foods. (Sorry Chef, I know you may be wincing about now, and it's not from chopping all those onions. A girl's gotta do what a girl's gotta do.)

Original Ingredients from MEAN . . .   TO "BITE ME!" CLEAN

Per Serving:	
Calories 662	Calories: 346
Protein: 41 g	Protein: 27g
Carbohydrates 55 g	Carbohydrates 42g
Fat 29 g	Fat: 8
Sat Fat: 13 g	Sat: 3
Chef's Ingredients:	BITE ME! Conversion:
2 cups fresh ricotta cheese	1/2 cup low-fat ricotta cheese, blended w 1 cup nonfat cottage cheese
8 ounces grated provolone	1 ounce grated provolone
8 ounces grated mozzarella	3 ounces reduced fat mozzarella
8 ounces grated Romano	1 ounce grated Romano
1 egg	2 egg whites
1/4 cup milk	1/4 cup nonfat milk
1 tablespoon chiffonade fresh basil leaves	Same
1 tablespoon chopped garlic	Same
Drizzle extra-virgin olive oil	Never drizzle, always measure. Here omit.
Salt	Omit.
Freshly ground black pepper	Same
1/2 pound grated Parmigiano-Reggiano	2 T Parmigiano-Reggiano
1 package no-cook lasagna noodles	1 package whole wheat lasagna noodles
Turkey Sausage Red Gravy:	
2 tablespoons olive oil	2 t nonstick cooking spray
2 pounds turkey sausage	1 Pkg lean ground turkey

Salt	Dash salt
Freshly ground black pepper	Same
2 cups finely chopped onions	Same
1/2 cup finely chopped celery	Same
1/2 cup finely chopped carrot	Add more vegetables, spinach
2 tablespoons chopped garlic	Same
(Homemade sauce recipe omitted)	One jar organic pasta sauce

Instructions: In a large saucepan over medium heat, coat lightly with olive oil or nonstick cooking spray. Add the ground turkey. Season with a dash of salt and pepper and mix well. Brown for 4 to 6 minutes, then drain. Add the onions, celery, carrots and spinach. Cook for 4 to 5 minutes or until the vegetables are soft. Blend into the turkey mixture and add tomato sauce. In a blender, mix the cottage cheese, ricotta, egg whites, and Parmigiano-Reggiano cheese. Layer glass pan with one cup of pasta sauce. Line with lasagna noodles. Add dollops of ricotta and cottage cheese mixture, and provolone and Romano sprinkles. Continue to layer with meat sauce. Bake at 350 degrees for 45 minutes.

JOURNALING FOODS

Journaling will provide insight into the quality of your foods as well as the calories. This is important because low quality foods are dense in calories, fat, sugar and sodium. High quality foods are typically lower in calories, providing a nutritional punch of essential vitamins, minerals and macronutrients. Calories matter too; you can eat too many calories of a healthy food and gain weight. So part of this equation is quality, the other is math.

Through the process of documenting your eating habits, you will uncover those daily behaviors that set you up for failure. Do you eat smart all week then binge on the weekends? Do you skip breakfast and snack until 2 AM? Do you go back for seconds when you don't need to? Are you eating mostly prepared, processed foods? Are you getting enough fruits and vegetables? You will glean the real truth about your habits, as long as you divulge the truth when writing down your foods.

It's interesting how far off our perception of our own habits differ from reality. Food journaling will expose our sabotaging indulgences, as well as bringing our good habits to light. I was at my daughter's school for an end of year luncheon for the 5th grade kids. One of the moms helping out was proud of herself for eating healthily during this lunch. She listed off all the foods, rice and beans, whole wheat tortillas, and fruit salad—which made a pretty good story–when in actuality I had watched her sabotage her good efforts with a deep fried Churro. Now I know this was an honest oversight on her part, and, curiously, omitted from her memory within five minutes of eating it. This elementary school lesson learned: Indulgences may taste good while you are enjoying them, but the satisfaction is short-lived, even so to the point where you can't even remember eating it an hour later.

Contrary to how it seems, journaling your foods doesn't take much time, and the wealth of knowledge you will learn will be invaluable. You don't need to journal for the rest of your life, just for a short time so you will have a realistic sense of what you are eating, portion size, and awareness of any undermining habits. You will in turn get the fastest results and will teach you how to "eyeball" your foods for the future.

Be sure to include the times for each meal, the quantity such as one cup or 3 ounces, as well as the specific food you ate. Don't forget to account for condiments as well, such as the creamer for your coffee or the oils used for cooking foods. You can use an online calorie counter, such as CalorieKing.com, to compile the calorie content of your favorite foods. Write it down in your journal and total the amount every day so you can see how much you are actually eating. Oftentimes restaurants will have nutrition information available as well; if so, you can find it on their website or at the establishment on menus.

So write it as you go, so you don't bury it into your subconscious. Your brain may not remember eating it but your thighs or gut most certainly will!

For a journal to print and use at home go to www.ToniJulian.com

SAMPLE JOURNAL

Date: Sunday, November 1ˢᵗ

Meal	Time	Amount	Food	Calories
Breakfast	7AM	1 cup	Pumpkin Oatmeal	250
		1	Orange	100
Morning Snack	10AM	1 small	Apple	240
		6	Raw Almonds	
		1	Hardboiled Egg	
Lunch	1PM	1 Serv	Edamame Salad	163
Afternoon Snack	4PM	1 cup	Yogurt	90
		1 med	Banana	100
		½ Serv	Whey Protein	120
Dinner	7PM	1 c	Cauliflower Soup	64
		1 Serv	Turkey with Eggplant	165
Evening Snack	9PM	1 Oatmeal	Cookie Shake	293
TOTALS				1585

Here are some journaling tips:

1. Be accurate; measure or weigh your food. You can buy an inexpensive food scale to weigh your lean meats. Are you eating three or eight ounces of fish? One half cup or one cup of rice? On numerous occasions my clients have reported to me they had a couple "handfuls of nuts." One portion is about ten almonds; how many in a couple of handfuls? It could be ten times that amount. Weigh and measure, it makes a difference!
2. Enter the times that you eat, account for breakfast, morning snack, lunch, afternoon snack, dinner, and after dinner snack. It will become evident if you are skipping meals, going many hours between eating, and overeating late at night.

3. The real revelation lies in the details so be certain to include the calories, carbohydrates, fat and protein. Add them up at the end of each day so you can see if you are getting a healthy balance. Typically 20% lean protein, 60% complex carbohydrates and 20% unsaturated, healthy fats are a good place to start. Each meal does not have to be perfectly balanced to those percentages, but you want to make sure you're getting what you need on a daily basis.

Tracking Calories and Macronutrients

Calculating macronutrients and calories can be cumbersome, and if you use the meal solutions in this book the work has been done for you. They are designed to streamline the process of estimating your calories for each meal. Every recipe has been accurately measured and prepared to ensure you are getting the most exacting accountability for nutrients and calories.

The Nutrition Profile information can be used in a number of ways depending upon the level of effort you want to invest:

1. *Ball parking*—paying attention to portion size and eating from the recipes you will have a general idea of the calories you are consuming
2. *Manual Tracking*—You may use your own journal, note paper or order one at www.ToniJulian.com.
3. *Calorie Management Software*—I often wonder where we would be without all the information available online. Calorie management programs are available to track online, or have simple look-up capabilities so you have instant access to the calorie and macronutrient information needed to manually journal. One of my favorites is Calorie King for look-up capabilities.
4. *Personal Calorie Management Tools*—If you'd really like to raise the bar, there are online services available that measure your activity level and your caloric intake. You wear an armband (hardware) and subscribe to an annual subscription to use their calorie tracking software. While this is not critical, it is a useful

tool but only as effective as you make it. Because I don't endorse products, you can Google "personal calorie management tools" or "online fitness tools" to research your options.

I wore a popular calorie-tracking armband for two years and it makes a great conversation starter. People would ask me what it was and for quite some time I sounded like a salesperson expounding on all the benefits, how it performed and how it works technically. It was exhausting. If I wear it occasionally now and get questions, I simply tell people I'm under house arrest and let them wonder what crime I've committed.

Any way you decide to go, be comforted by the fact that you won't need to wear an armband or log your foods forever. I tracked my foods for a period of about two years longer than needed, however, and I have learned exactly how much food I need every day, how much to eat at each meal, how often to eat, which foods are wholesome and clean, and I don't really need to think much about it. I no longer need to weigh and measure my foods; I can visualize the amount from practicing. I can manipulate my weight up or down depending on whether I am leaning down temporarily to prepare for a competition, or need to slightly increase my caloric intake with increased activity. Once you learn how to eat, it's important not to obsess about it.

NewsBite: Take charge of portion control

Ever pick up a box of cereal, even a healthy one, and before you know it, it's half gone? Those calories can really add up! Here's a tip: as soon as you buy it measure out all the portions and put ONE portion each in a zip lock bag, then put all the baggies back in the original container. When you want to reach for a snack, or if you're on the go, just take ONE bag and that's it. You don't have to think about it, which is what gets us into the inadvertent overeating to begin with.

CHAPTER 16

THE EIGHT WEEK "BITE ME!" CHALLENGE

"There are no ugly women, only lazy ones."
~Helena Rubenstein

Helena, an entrepreneur, was one of the most alluring women of her time. She was no natural beauty, but she knew how to take care of herself and it showed. What better way is there to motivate people to take impeccable care of themselves through fitness and eating healthy, other than to present a challenge?

This section is in celebration of the women who whole-heartedly participated in the very first BITE ME! Challenge. As soon as this book became available, our clients were so enthusiastic, several of them wanted to be put to the test. Meet Victoria, Heather, Jo Ann, Bonnie, Debbie and Patti.

The ultimate goal: to see who could transform their body the most in eight weeks, eating primarily from the recipes in this book, and incorporating the guidelines for clean eating habits. (Participants, as well as all readers of this book, are encouraged to experiment with the recipes and substitute a variety of other healthy, whole foods to provide a full spectrum of nutrients.)

The participants represented a realistic cross-section of differing age ranges, body types, and fitness levels; the majority of them were current participants of The Booty Club; our outdoor personalized training program which combines a unique combination of cardiovascular and resistance training exercises, in a fun, supportive and highly personalized environment.

Getting Dunked!

To kick off our eight-week challenge, everyone participated in a hydrostatic immersion test to establish an accurate and measurable body fat benchmark. Also known as an underwater "dunk," this test measures the actual amount of body fat and lean muscle mass based on the concept that fat is more buoyant than its denser counterpart, muscle. A report is then generated detailing specific results, such as the total body fat and lean mass in pounds, and it provides a percentage. As an example, a typical de-conditioned and slightly overweight woman in her 40's could be around 30%, which means nearly 1/3 of her body weight is fat and the rest is lean mass—whereas a female athlete may be as low as 15% body fat, or even lower. *(It is important to note that we all need body fat for survival: for energy storage and to cushion our internal organs. See a professional to determine your healthy goal!)*

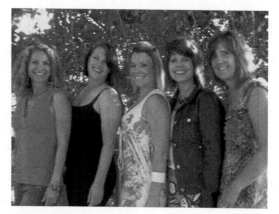

A "benchmark" picture of some of the BITE ME! Challenge contenders, starting from left to right, Toni Guiliani-Apgar, and participants Victoria Pearce-Kelso, Heather Buchholz, Jo Ann Lauer, and Patti Keating.

The most phenomenal part of this program is to watch the results. It's a well-known fact: 95% of all people who take weight off through dieting gain their weight back, and then some, within the first year. A lifestyle change is incremental progress, which yields permanent results. The goal is to gain muscle and lose fat over time. The results of the top three BITE ME! Challenge contestants all demonstrate that the results are for life! You will see their benchmarks, and now over one year later their results are even more phenomenal. Eat correctly and you will be rewarded!

CONTESTANT RESULTS

2009 SPRING CHALLENGE

I am so proud of the women who accept the challenge because every one of them made a shift in the right direction. Our group of seven women collectively lost a total of 63 pounds in eight weeks! As you may know, on an average, we gain about a pound of fat per year, and we lose muscle mass due to de-conditioning. It is admirable to step up to the challenge, it is commendable to maintain; it is exceptional to actually reverse the trend!

It was a close competition; in our first Spring Challenge our top three contenders lost nearly equivalent amounts of fat. However, our first place winner not only held onto her existing muscle mass, but actually gained some in the process.

First Place "BITE ME!" Challenge Winner: Patti Keating

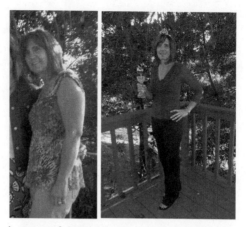

Patti, at the start of the challenge—then only eight weeks later in a progress photo—is the winner of the BITE ME! Challenge donning her tiara and golden disco ball award (she always wanted to win the "Dancing with the Stars" award).

Patti shared with me her experience in adopting these lifestyle changes. Her toughest challenge as a stylist and owner of a popular salon, City Savvy in Campbell, is that she is on her feet all day and has difficulty eating at regular intervals while juggling client appointments.

What makes Patti's achievement particularly commendable is that she is a breast cancer survivor, and had not incorporated an exercise regimen after her reconstructive surgery. Over a year ago she joined the aabs**Booty**Club™, has embraced an entirely clean way of eating, and quit drinking alcohol. She has learned to take impeccable care of herself, in spite of life's obstacles.

My observation is that her success comes from doing a tremendous job of experimenting with the recipes in this book; she sets aside time one day each week to prepare her meals so she and her family always have healthy options. Because she adopted the lifestyle changes, she now brings healthy snacks, like muffins, protein shakes, and prepared chicken, quinoa and veggies to keep her energized throughout the day. Patti is amazed at how well she feels and told me an added benefit is that her husband unexpectedly lost his love handles in the process! Oh la la! Congratulations, Patti!

Patti's Stats

Age 55, Salon Owner/Stylist

Success: One Year and Later	During the 8-week Challenge	Overall
Body Composition Changed:	4.3%	11%
Starting Body Fat %:	30.7%	
Ending Body Fat %:	25.0%	9.6%
Total Fat Loss in Pounds	10	15.4
Muscle Gain	1	2.6

Second Place Winner
Debbie Butera

Age: 54
Occupation: Sales Associate

Debbie epitomizes the progress that I prefer to see in our challengers. She has come a long way, and as a mom with three daughters and an busy lifestyle, she strives to be consistent amidst life's social temptations. When a large part of the population gains their weight back within the first year, Debbie wholeheartedly accepted this program as incremental changes, and her accomplishments are consistent with her efforts.

Success: One Year and Later	During the 8-week Challenge	Overall
Body Composition Changed:	4.1%	4.8%
Starting Body Fat %:	30.8	
Ending Body Fat %:	26.7	26%

Total Fat Loss in Pounds	9.5	10.8
Muscle Gain	1.5	3.8%

Third Place Winner
Heather Buchholz

Age: 30
Occupation: Service Sales

Success:	**During the 8-week Challenge**	**Overall**
One Year and Later		
Body Composition Changed:		
Starting Body Fat %:	21.5	
Ending Body Fat %:	19.0	14.9
Total Fat Loss in Pounds	8.5	10.5
Muscle Gain—	3.4	4

One year later: 14.9%

2011 Winter Challenge

First Place Winner
Eda Vincenzini

Another exceptional first place winner is Eda. She had struggled with her weight for a couple of years. Initially, she had lost 70 pounds through a medically supervised supplement diet, but had gained every ounce right back. Being a nurse, she was under extreme stress at work and found it challenging to avoid sugar, indulging in sweets on a daily basis. Eda was participating in our winter challenge when unfortunately, while skiing she broke her ankle. I thought most certainly we should adjust her goals to maintenance mode given her immobility. What is most remarkable is that not only did Eda avoid gaining weight, but she changed her body composition by 5.4 percent with a broken ankle! She changed her undermining habits to healthy ones, focusing entirely on eating from this book and the payoff was enormous. Congratulations Eda!

Success:	During the 8-week Challenge
Body Composition Changed:	5.4%
Starting Body Fat:	37.7%
Ending Body Fat:	32.3%
Total Fat Loss in Pounds:	12.4
Muscle Gain:	2.9

Second Place Winner

Wendy Crayton
Success:	During the 8-week Challenge
Body Composition Changed:	5.2%
Starting Body Fat:	31.7%
Ending Body Fat:	24.9%
Total Fat Loss in Pounds:	12.0
Muscle Gain:—	.1

Spring 2010 Challenge

First Place Winner
Terri-Lynn Riegler, Age 48

Body Composition Changed:	6.3%
Starting Body Fat:	28%
Ending Body Fat:	21.7%
Total Fat Loss in Pounds:	10.0
Muscle Gain:	5.5

Here's Terri's story!

"I visited the aabs Lifestyle and Fitness Coaching site and started to read a bit about Toni and how she started her venture into the world of fitness and health. As I was reading her story of reinventing herself at 50, I can clearly see that Toni is just as real as anyone else and had experienced the same things in life that most of us had experienced as well. The difference being, she had taken control of her life, her health her well being and gradually reinvented herself. She wasn't offering up some miracle weight loss program; "lose 10 pounds in a week" or gimmicks of that nature. Something we all tend to fall prey to, only to find we have wasted our money and have seen little to no results in these "Quick" weight loss scams, or diets that set you up for failure. Toni's approach is very realistic and very attainable.

I am nearly 48 years old and have experienced my share of health issues since 2003. With having Sarcoidosis; (resulting in the removal of ½ of a lung), High Blood Pressure, Boarder Diabetic and High Cholesterol, I knew I needed to do something for my benefit and to get off the various medications I have been taking, so I purchased Toni's "BITE-ME" lifestyle change book online and made a few of the recipe. I noticed that I was losing some weight. (At this time, I weighed in between 153—156 and could never seem to get out of that 150 zone). I had inquired about the "aabs**Booty**Club™" and Toni was able to put together another class that was convenient so I joined! I have done the gym routine, I own many workout DVD's, but eventually I would either lose interest, or think up some excuse in my head why I didn't need to take 45 minutes a few days a week to work out. The Booty Club was much different and I really enjoyed my workout sessions, even though they were at 6 am! The morning drive to the park was very relaxing, the fresh air in the morning . . . perfect way to start the day and feel accomplished! The group was a lot of fun and all very encouraging. After about a month, my boyfriend had commented on how much happier I had become and he started seeing subtle changes in my body. He attributed the change to my workouts.

I hired Toni for weekly lifestyle coaching sessions to review my eating habits. I thought I was always a healthy eater, but Toni had pointed out things that I never really considered was causing my "Muffin Top" to hang around. When we first sat down to go over foods I would eat during the day, I was barely consuming 950-1000 calories per day, causing my body to hang on to the fat. During the course of the 8 week challenge, I had noticed my stomach was slimming, my clothes were fitting loose (I was wearing between a size 8-9). My boyfriend noticed I was changing more and more. He had taken me clothes shopping because my clothes were getting too big. I was amazed to find that I was able to wear a size 6!

Since completing the challenge, I have made my goal of 135 lbs. And still buying smaller clothes! I recently took a trip to Arizona to visit family. I was greeted with "WOW" where did you go? You look great! It was obvious I had lost weight and made healthy changes. To date, I maintain my healthy eating habits and I limit my alcohol intake. I will continue to incorporate the recipes from Toni's book into my daily life.

Toni was and still is very encouraging and always gives praise. Her genuine sincerity, kind spirit and never ending encouragement speak volumes. This program is definitely a life changing experience!

Are You Ready for the Challenge?

"If you fail to plan then you are planning to fail." ~ Unknown Author
Let's talk about YOU! Are you ready to take on the challenge? Have you reached the point where you know in your heart it's time to feel better? Looking better on the outside is a direct reflection of taking care of yourself from the inside-out. I'm fairly sure I heard an enthusiastic "YES!" from you. All right, then, it's time to light a fire under your booty . . . .

Let's start with feeling better and learning how to improve your eating habits, adopting healthier lifestyles first. Once you begin to feel better, then the weight WILL begin to come off. Let's NOT pay homage to the scale-God each morning, praying that we do not have to pay for our sinful indulgences the night before. Instead, let's start by focusing on making healthier choices and identifying ONE way you sabotage yourself. Ask yourself, "What would be a better choice?" Then, be prepared with an answer, and have that new and healthier food at hand. Boot your old convenience food fixes to the curb and substitute it with a clean-eating option. Weigh yourself only once each week.

Take Three Easy Steps!

STEP ONE: Be prepared! Pick a few recipes from this book to begin with. As an example, Purely Pumpkin Oatmeal for breakfast, Apple-Carrot Bran Muffins for meal time snacks, the Yummy Yam Fries or Turkey Bean Stew for lunches or dinners. You can select any recipe and eat it any time of the day, just be sure to spread the calories out evenly into 5 or 6 small meals throughout the day. Make sure to follow the 10 Quick Tips for Clean Eating.

STEP TWO: Shop for your groceries a day or two in advance, then, schedule a two to three hour block of time to make all the meals you selected. As you get more accustomed to the recipes, it will take less preparation time. Partition your foods into individual servings and freeze what you think you will not eat over the next few days. Whenever you're hungry, you'll have a plan to eat a healthy food. Replace your less than optimum convenience foods with a wholesome, clean food and you will be satisfied. You will also be making a healthy choice by being proactive and being prepared! Starving and on the go? Have a BITE ME! Banana-Nut muffin . . . yummy!

STEP THREE; Lose weight in a healthy way, S-L-O-W-L-Y, to ensure these are in fact lifestyle changes, and not a restrictive diet. If weight loss is your goal, please don't starve yourself. You will only lose muscle if you go too quickly which will decrease your metabolism. You will keep the weight off; you will not feel deprived, but satisfied. A good target is a 500 calorie deficit each day, but never to go below 1200 to ensure proper nutrition. This deficit should result in a one pound loss over a week, depending upon how many calories you are burning each day. Doesn't sound like much? Grab a pound of butter out of your refrigerator and put it on the counter.

Now imagine that one pound melting off your thighs over the next week. It may not seem like much, but it is significant if you can put a visual behind what you are really doing. Keep your calories in a healthy range, and start moving. Walking, hiking, cycling . . . anything that will help you burn additional calories adds to your success.

If your calories are too low, your body will want to hold on to the fat. Retrain it by letting it know it will have nutrients coming in every few hours though eating your clean-eating meals.

Perhaps you're one of those people who survive on 1200 a day or less. Slowly bring up your calories in 200-calorie increments. As an example: consume 1400 calories a day for two weeks (your starting, typical caloric intake), then 1600 for two weeks, then 1800 for two weeks. Surprisingly, all of my clients who are re-taught how to eat do not gain any weight on this plan, they maintain. Once your calories are in line with your actual expenditure, then your metabolism has been re-trained. Only then can you reduce your calories to drop weight. Clients are occasionally frustrated with having to "wait" to start losing weight, but it is progress and a critical part of ensuring you get the nutrients you need.

I have heard of nutritionists or doctors putting some of my clients on an 800 calorie per day weight loss plan and it frankly stupefies me. It leaves them with no place to go and feeling deprived and cranky. Even worse, it is not sustainable so the majority of people gain weight their back after all that hard work.

If your goal is to tone, sculpt or become more cut, add weight resistance exercises. This could mean your own body weight, dumbbells or hiring a personal trainer at the gym. Or if you are in our neck of the woods, join our Booty Club for supportive and fun outdoor personalized training!

And please do not get overly hung up on the scale. If you are gaining muscle, and losing fat, you may not see a reduction in scale weight right away. However you will be more toned, slowly increasing your metabolism in the process.

FOR BEST RESULTS

The best results come when you have support. Illicit the help of a friend or your family and join the BITE ME! Challenge together.

Encouragement goes a long way and we all know . . . it takes a village. Good luck! Stay healthy and above all, persevere!

FREE 8 Week BITE ME! Challenge Contest

Go to www.ToniJulian.com to receive your application. There are no hidden costs, subscriptions or obligations.

Send your progress picture at the 8 week mark, along with a summary of how you achieved your goals and which aspects of this program most contributed to your success. One first place winner will be selected at the first of every month.

PAY IT FORWARD

In keeping with the philosophy of this book, you won't be able to retire on millions of dollars of prize money. If you didn't get the message earlier, you should be doing this for you! Instead, help your friends and loved ones as a first place winner by sharing your success. Pay it forward by gifting free 90-minute life coaching sessions with Toni Julian to three people (not including yourself) who you know will benefit. They will not only have your support, but also the extra professional direction to get them started on their new journey! As the top placing contender, you will be featured on the website along with your top two competitors. Visit www.ToniJulian.com for more details!

Chapter 17

Trouble-Shooting Guide

If Microsoft Windows has a trouble shooting guide, your body should too! This chapter is for those who have weight loss goals and feel they've given this program a good shot, but they are not seeing a reduction in their scale weight.

First, keep in mind if you were on an upward weight-gaining trend, and if you've found you have not continued to gain weight but have leveled out, that is progress in itself. You can attribute your eating and fitness regimen to maintaining your weight. Once you have reached your goals, your current habits and behaviors will work for you in your maintenance mode in the future.

Secondly, if you are not losing "scale weight" and your clothes fit better than they have before, it is highly likely you have gained muscle and lost fast. Remember fat takes up to three times the volume of muscle pound for pound.

Below are the most common reasons people may not make as much progress as they would like:

1. Not keeping accurate food journals
   Journaling your foods for a short time, and measuring or weighing will give you insight into portion control and caloric intake. The

most common reason people aren't making progress is they are underestimating the calories they are consuming. It's a learning experience so review the chapter on journaling if you haven't already done so.

2. Undiagnosed medical conditions

   Be sure to have your thyroid and other hormones checked by a physician or OB/GYN. You need to be aware of hormonal imbalances as they can work against you. If you are post menopausal, allow yourself more time to see changes; unfortunately it takes longer once your body has begun to change.

3. Not eating enough calories

   You may be under-eating which won't allow you to re-set your metabolism. Be sure to enough small, frequent meals throughout the day.

4. Treating this program as a diet

   If you have been severely restricting calories or particular food items, you may be feeling deprived which is just setting you up for failure. Implement one change at a time, a change that is a lifestyle change that is sustainable for life. Diets fail, and so will you if you look at this as one.

5. Refusing to let go of destructive social habits

   Your body will not change, if you do not change your behavior around eating and exercise. An entire weeks' worth of "being good" can unravel if you are cheating on the weekends. Consistent eating habits are imperative to your success. Think about the math; if you are eating at a 300 calorie deficit each day, you will likely lose 2/3's of a pound each week, which is equivalent to 2100 calories. You think you've done great! Now you can go to a party and eat dip, chips, dessert, two margaritas and an entrée. You've not only sabotaged your whole week, you've exceeded your deficit and added extra sodium. Your weight will probably be up a couple of pounds by Monday. Party after you've met your goals, it's not the end of the world.

6. Not cooking for yourself

   My fantasy is to have someone in the house chopping all my fruits and vegetables so I can indulge in them at a whim. Some of my clients are fortunate to have amazing husbands that cook! In fact they do all the cooking for all the meals, however the trade off is that unless they follow or modify their recipes to the guidelines in this book, you are really not eating as clean as you need to. And yes, that is enough to sabotage your best efforts. Two of my clients' husbands are professional chefs and getting them to stop layering every technique with oil or butter is challenging. Take control over what is going into your mouth if you want results.

If you feel you need additional help, go to www.ToniJulian.com for information on private or group nutrition and lifestyle coaching sessions with Toni Julian.

CHAPTER 18

Q& A

How does one maintain the motivation and focus to keep going on with their new lifestyle and meal plan? I battle with this every day. Norma C., Fresno, CA

That is a superb question and also gives me insight into where you are currently. If it feels like a "battle" for you then we need to adjust your goals to make it suit your lifestyle and not be so challenging. People typically feel this way when the plan is activated as a diet—that is, too many changes at once—and it feels restrictive on a daily basis and hard to achieve. The main difference between a LIFESTYLE CHANGE and a DIET is SUSTAINABILITY. For now, your goal should be to maintain as you are going through additional challenges in your life. Maintenance is still a great goal; it takes work to achieve and is appropriate when life gets rough. Let's work on modifying your short-term objectives and make it more manageable for you.

I'm 77, have diabetes, and usually don't eat until the afternoon. I'm still not hungry around 4PM but eat because I think I should. Why can I go most of the day without eating and not feel hungry or affected? ~ Lois, Jalisco, Mexico

You are so accustomed to going long stretches without eating; your body has shut off its appetite mechanism. If after 3 or 4 hours after eating, you are still not hungry, eat half of a meal. Especially with breakfast, eat something very small, such as a quarter of a protein bar or one egg, to awaken your appetite. With diabetes, you need to be especially careful not to skip meals. Lower the overall glycemic load by balancing each meal with protein, low glycemic index complex carbohydrates and healthy fats, such as olive oil, avocado, nuts and seeds. It goes without saying, be sure to consult your doctor in regards to any medical issues or diseases.

For the recipes, can I substitute some of my own ingredients?
Colleen, San Jose, CA

Absolutely! You are encouraged to swap out ingredients to ensure greater variety and therefore additional nutrients in your diet. Exchange any vegetable for another vegetable, lean meat for another source of lean protein, etc. For example, instead of the ground turkey in the Turkey Bean Soup, you can use cubed or shredded chicken or tofu if you are vegan. In place of applesauce in a muffin, add chopped apples or a ripe banana. I encourage you to experiment, add as many colors to your plate as possible and have fun with your food.

I never know what to eat after a workout. Any suggestions? Wendy, San Jose, CA

The same thing you would eat for every other meal: a balance of lean protein, complex carbohydrates and healthy fats.

By the time I get off work and go to the gym, its 9:00pm. What is the latest at night that I should eat? Renee R., San Jose, CA

I think the question behind your question is, "How late can I eat without gaining weight?" because of the association with eating late at night and weight gain. In the fitness industry, there are mixed beliefs, most likely because there are so many variables. It depends on your calorie deficit for that day; if you have eaten fewer calories than you have burned and feel hungry before bed, a light snack is in order. Try to keep it to mostly protein so your muscles can use it to repair overnight—perhaps some nonfat yogurt with a few almonds. Snacking at night becomes an issue if you have already consumed enough calories to break even, and you add additional calories late into the evening, whether high quality food or not. Your body does not require these and the extra energy is converted to fat for future use.

What are your thoughts on energy drinks? Charles L., San Jose, CA My question to you would be why do you feel you need them? If you keep your body in homeostasis, your blood sugar regulated, through sleep and eating correctly, your body would be functioning optimally and you would not need to supplement through the use of stimulants, such as caffeine. Energy drinks amongst teens and older is becoming a problem, especially when combined with alcohol. The stimulant creates a false sense of being in control and does not diminish the effect of the alcohol. Energy drinks are considered supplements, and any claims made by these companies are not evaluated by the FDA. My advice: avoid them entirely and rely on fueling your body in a balanced way.

How do I know how many calories I am burning every day? Anna B., Los Gatos, CA

There are several ways to go about estimating what you burn—including BMR formulas, food journaling, metabolism testing and online calorie and exercise tracking software.

BMR Formula

The first method to estimate is through a formula –which I realize is a lot of math but worth the time if you really want to know.
You must start with your BMR or Basil Metabolic Rate, which is the energy expended while at complete rest. Out of the totally energy expended in a day, roughly 70% is due to supporting our basil life process. Another 20% typically comes from physical activity, and the remaining 10% is from the energy required to digest food.

BMR Formula for Women: BMR = 655 + (4.35 x weight in pounds) + (4.7 x height in inches)—(4.7 x age in years)

For example, if you're a 46 year old woman, weighing 148 pounds and are 5' 3" in height, here's how it works:

BMR= 655 + (4.35 x 148) + (4.7 x 63)—(4.7 x 46) = 1378 calories per day

To take it a step further and estimate how many total calories you may burn in a 24-hour period:

1378 divided by .7 (to calculate total calories) = 1969

BMR:	70%	1378
Activity:	20%	394
Digestion:	10%	197

Total Estimated Calories per Day: 1969

If you are physically active, and as an example, work out for an hour, you would add approximately 300 calories to the total. This method provides a good baseline.

BMR Formula for Men:
BMR = 66 + (6.23 x weight in pounds) + (12.7 x height in inches)—(6.8 x age in year)

Example for a man, age 35, weighing 185 and 5' 11" is below
BMR= 655 + (4.35 x 148) + (4.7 x 63)—(4.7 x 46) = 1628 calories per day

Food Journaling

Day 1: Weigh yourself first thing in the morning without clothes and before a meal or water. Measure and write down the foods you eat every meal and add up the calories at the end of each day.

Days 2-7: Continue food journaling.

Day 8: Weigh yourself using the same method as on day 1. If you have lost one pound, this means that you were at a 3500 calorie deficit for the week. Add up your daily journal calorie totals for the week, and add the 3500 calories. Divide that by 7 for your daily average and that is roughly what you burn every day. Use the same method if you have gained weight, only subtract the calories from your weekly total and divide by 7.

(Pounds Lost) x (3500 calories per pound) divided by (7 days of the week) = calorie deficit per day

I've been dealing with digestive issues, and especially have problems with wheat and gluten. Can you make a recommendation for what would help me? Robbie T., San Jose, CA

Gluten sensitivity and related digestive issues are becoming more prevalent, and it's not because there are new cases, but because only 95% of Celiac Disease (toxic reaction to gluten, the protein found in wheat) has been diagnosed in this country so the awareness has increased. There has been little research and education in this area until recently because there is no pharmacological cure, purely a nutritional solution. Sticking to unprocessed foods that you prepare yourself will give you the best relief and if you are diligent about it, and will allow the villi in your small intestine to heal. Some people can handle some level of gluten and others become severely ill with only trace amounts. Consistency is the key. Probiotics can help by providing healthy bacteria for your intestines. Note: new processed gluten-free foods arrive on the market daily, although, just because it is gluten free, it does not mean it is healthy for you as it may be loaded with highly processed starches, sugars and fat. The tools in this book will help you build a strong nutritional foundation, and if you are consistent and compliant while eliminating gluten, you will minimize Celiac's damaging effects. You can substitute gluten-free versions of foods, such as Bob's Red Mill Gluten-Free Oats in place of regular oats, Bob's Mighty Tasty Cereal in place of bread crumbs or oat bran, and organic gluten-free chicken broth in place of the Swanson's. Whole Foods has an enormous selection of gluten-free foods, Trader Joe's has a few as well.

Acknowledgements and Gratitude

To my Lifestyle Coaching and aabs**Booty**Club™ clients; witnessing them making great strides in transforming their bodies; their feedback and success, has been invaluable. They've allowed me to take an intimate accounting of their lives, and their candidness and open-minded attitudes have led me to develop great respect for them. To all my clients, an enormous "Thank you!"

To Adam, my personal trainer who helped guide me through my personal fitness journey, where I could find my true purpose helping others do the same.

To my team of talented doctors, Dr. Margaret Mahoney, Dr. Samir Sharma, Dr. Amy Gonsier, Dr. Ken Miller, Dr. Pamela Nomura, Dr. Eugene Della Maggiore, and Dr. Robert Millard; all who helped get me through some tumultuous times, and Dr. Samual Ballon, my Gynecological Oncologist to whom I owe so much, and most especially Dr. David Cahn, who for the last 20 years has given out more hugs than prescriptions. May you never retire!

To my friend Charlie who said, "If you want to help more people, write a book," so I did.

To my best friends, Jan, Valerie, Kara, Patti and Dee Dee, and in spirit, Barb; there is no replacement in my life for any of you.

And most importantly, to my supportive family; my handsome and brilliant husband who loves me unconditionally and helps ground me, to our kids who I am so proud of for their individual gifts, to my brother who brings levity to my life, to my giving sister, to my father, who is uniquely witty, bright, and taught me how to be a good person, and finally, to my mom who brought me into this world and shared her gifts of creativity and free-spirit. I got the best of both from them.

Thank you to everyone who has been waiting patiently for my book. If I could walk and type at the same time it would have been less of a wait!